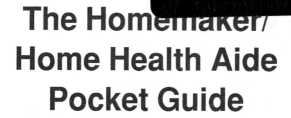

The Homemaker/ Home Health Aide Pocket Guide

Elana Zucker R.N., M.S.N

Vice President
Patient Services Operations
Overlook Hospital
Summit, New Jersey

Prentice Hall Career & Technology
Englewood Cliffs, New Jersey 07632

Library of Congress Cataloging-in-Publication Data

Zucker, Elana D., (date)
   The homemaker/home health aide pocket guide / Elana Zucker.
     p.   cm.
   "A Brady Book."
   Companion volume to: Being a homemaker/home health aide / Elana D.
Zucker, editor. 1988
   ISBN 0-89303-691-9
   1. Home health aides—Handbooks, manuals, etc. 2. Home care
services—Handbooks, manuals, etc. 3. Home nursing—Handbooks,
manuals, etc. I. Being a homemaker/home health aide. II. Title.
   [DNLM: 1. Home Care Services—handbooks. WY 39 Z94h]
RA645.3.Z826 1990
649.8—dc20
DNLM/DLC
for Library of Congress   89-23197
                                      CIP

Editorial/production supervision
  and page layout: PATRICK WALSH
  Cover Design: EDSAL ENTERPRISES
  Manufacturing Buyer: DAVID DICKEY

 © 1990 Prentice-Hall, Inc.
A Simon & Schuster Company
Englewood Cliffs, New Jersey 07632

Printed in the United States of America

10 9 8

ISBN 0-89303-691-9

Prentice-Hall International (UK) Limited, *London*
Prentice-Hall of Australia Pty. Limited, *Sydney*
Prentice-Hall Canada, Inc., *Toronto*
Prentice-Hall Hispanoamericana, S.A., *Mexico*
Prentice-Hall of India Private Limited, *New Delhi*
Prentice-Hall of Japan, Inc., *Tokyo*
Simon & Schuster Asia Pte. Ltd., *Singapore*
Editora Prentice-Hall do Brasil, Ltda., *Rio de Janeiro*

Contents

Preface

The Homemaker/Home Health Aide Pocket Guide has been created as a reference for you to use as you care for your client. Many times, while performing your duties, you have a question or want to check your information; this book is designed for those quick reviews. It can also be used when you are planning care and want to be sure that all important points have been covered in your plan, or as a handy quick reference when you want to review a specific idea you had learned in class. For ease, all clients are referred to as "he" and all homemaker/home health aides are referred to as "she." This is purely an editorial prerogative.

Keeping in mind that your most important task is caring for your client, the content is arranged for easy quick reference. Tables, lists, and illustrations are used throughout. Procedures have been shortened to reflect the fact that those people using the book will all be experienced health-care workers. Should more complete explanation be needed, you are referred to the text book, *Being a Homemaker/Home Health Aide*, Second Edition.

You are encouraged to familiarize yourself with the layout of the book so that you will be able to find the information quickly. Write in the book and make notes. Use the book as a teaching tool for your clients. Use it as a quick review as you provide care.

Elana Zucker

Introduction

YOUR RESPONSIBILITY AS AN EMPLOYEE OF A HOME CARE AGENCY

It is your responsibility to perform the tasks you are assigned to the best of your ability. Perform *only* those tasks that are part of your assignment. If you do not know a procedure or have a question be sure to *ask*! You are expected to care for the clients in a thoughtful, respectful, and considerate manner. It is also expected that you will share your ideas, thoughts, and observations with your supervisor and fellow employees.

You will be expected to use many different pieces of equipment. Be sure you are familiar with each one. If you do not know how to use a piece of equipment safely and easily be sure to *ask*! Sometimes you may need to ask the client, sometimes you will ask a family member, and sometimes you will ask your supervisor. It is important to ask for instructions before you use the equipment so that you do not harm the client or yourself.

When you receive your assignment ask your supervisor the following:

- What equipment is needed for the client's care?
- Who will obtain the needed equipment? Will the family buy it? Will the nurse bring it? Will it be delivered?
- Are the necessary tools and equipment to keep the house clean available? Will the family purchase any needed equipment or supplies?

Try to use equipment and supplies that are already in the house. The client and his family are used to these. If you have tried to use the equipment and supplies that have been provided and you still find that you need something, discuss this with your supervisor. She may have suggestions for ways in which you can improvise or ways in which the equipment or supplies you require can be obtained. Keep in mind that one of your responsibilities is to set up the client's care so that he can continue it on his own when you leave. Your use of equipment and supplies that are familiar to him is part of this process.

YOUR RESPONSIBILITIES AS A HOMEMAKER/ HOME HEALTH AIDE

You are expected to be familiar with your job description. This includes understanding what your role is within the agency and as part of the home care team. It is your responsibility to perform the assigned tasks to the best of your ability. You are to perform *only* those tasks that are part of your assignment.

When you first meet the client and the other members of his household, remember that you are a stranger to them. There will be a period of time when you will all have to get to know one another. Helpful hints to make this period easier are:

- *Wear your uniform.* This identifies you as a member of the health team.
- *Wear your name pin.* This tells the family that you are who you say you are.
- *Introduce yourself.* Write down your name and the name of your agency if the client cannot remember them. Write down the telephone number that the client can call to ask questions or to reach you or your supervisor.
- *Discuss with the client and his family what you can do and what you cannot do.* Tell them how long you will be there. Involve the client and his family in the plan of care. Assure them that you will structure your care so that the client is comfortable.
- *Answer the client's questions.* Be honest. If he asks for information you do not have or are not supposed to discuss, you might say, "I do not have the answer now, but I will get you the information." Then call your supervisor and work out a response for the client. Be sure to give the client an answer the next time you see him, and be sure it is an honest one. Do not lie because the client may never trust you again.

YOUR NEEDS AS A HOMEMAKER/HOME HEALTH AIDE

It is important that you meet your needs as a person and as a homemaker/home health aide, but not at the expense of your client. There are many times when you will have to put aside your needs until you leave your client. When you feel you can no longer do this, speak to your supervisor. As you care for your client, ask yourself:

- Are you meeting your needs or your client's needs?

- Do you perform a procedure with the client because he enjoys having you help or do you feel you *must* do it?
- Does helping a client become independent make you feel good or useless?

1

Communication Skills

HOW DO WE COMMUNICATE?

Communication means exchanging information with others. People let others know how they feel or what they think all day and even during the night. Communication is necessary so people can function together.

When you are working in peoples' homes, it is important that *their* opinions and feelings be the ones that shape the care and activity in the home. If you are asked for your opinion and it is different from your client's, you might say, "This is your house and here it is more important how you feel about this situation than how I feel."

Verbal communication takes place when people speak to each other. The tone of voice, the speed of the conversation, and the word patterns all serve to tell something about the speaker.

Writing and drawing are forms of *written communication*. The neatness of the writing and the choice of words indicate how the writer views the subject.

Nonverbal communication is made up by the way in which we hold our bodies, the facial expressions we use, our general appearance, eye contact, hand movements, and the way in which we touch others.

A GOOD LISTENER IS

- *A careful listener.* Listen to what is said, what is not said, to the speaker's choice of words, and to the tone of voice.
- *Sensitive.* Respect the client's moods. There are times when a person does not wish to speak.
- *Courteous.* Be courteous to your client and to your fellow workers. Give others a chance to express their ideas without being interrupted. Say everything in the nicest way you know.
- *In control of her emotions.* If you feel like making a rude or nasty remark, don't do it! If a client or family member is rude or difficult to deal with, offer to listen to the client or get another member of the health care team to help with the problem. Answering in a rude manner will not help.
- *Receptive to constructive criticism.* Accept suggestions from your supervisor, fellow workers, and your client or his family. If you do not agree with the suggestions, discuss the criticism; don't discuss the person who made them.
- *Truthful to the client.* The client may ask you a question about his doctor or the doctor's diagnosis. *Do not lie to the client!* Do not tell the client you do not know something when you should be aware of the information. If you lie, the client may find out and never trust you again. It is no shame to say you do not have the information readily at hand. But if you say you do not know, you close the conversation. Tell the client you

will get the answer. Then call your supervisor to discuss the question and plan an answer. When you promise to get an answer for a client, do it!

FAMILY AND VISITORS

A client usually feels better when he knows family and friends are concerned and make an effort to visit. Visitors may be worried and upset over the illness of your client. Visitors may need your kindness and patience. They may need to be instructed as to how to act with your client and what to expect during the visit. You may have to help visitors make the most of their visit without tiring your client. You may tactfully have to suggest that the visitors leave so your client can rest.

- Try not to get involved in family affairs. Never take sides in an argument.
- If visitors ask questions you cannot or do not feel are proper to answer, tell them you will get the information. Then contact your supervisor to discuss the questions and plan the answer.
- If visitors or family members ask how they may help, give suggestions.
- Visitors may try to give you orders. Be open about your responsibilities. Explain that your supervisor sets up the plan of care and you will discuss changes with her.
- Listen to family and visitors. Some of their suggestions may help you. They may tell you things about your client that will help you understand him better. Ask these family members to be a part of the care of the client. Often they will have to assume the care when you are no longer in the home. This is a perfect time for them to learn.

- Report the family dynamics that you observe. These can be very helpful to your supervisor in planning the care of your client.

CLIENT OBSERVATION: RECORDING AND REPORTING

Observe the client during all your contacts such as bathing, bed making, meal times, and exercise time.

Subjective reporting: giving your opinion about something or what you think might be the case.

Objective reporting: reporting exactly what you observe. That is, reporting what you see, smell, hear, or feel.

General information: changes in the environment, the family dynamics, and visitors.

Specific information: observations you have made about the client.

When you receive your assignment ask:

- Is there a special time for me to call the office?
- Is there a special number to reach my supervisor?
- If my supervisor is not in the office, who will help me?
- Can I call from the client's house? If not, where is the nearest phone?
- What information does the agency give by telephone and what is given in writing?
- What type of information should be reported verbally and what should be written?
- What is the correct mailing address of the office?
- What is correct amount of postage to use?

What Do You Report?

Know what information must be telephoned to your supervisor and what information is to be sent by mail. It is important for you to discuss with your supervisor the type of information you should report. Reporting your observations protects you from being held responsible for a possible mistake. When you communicate to another member of the health team, you should:

- Be sure of your information.
- Have complete information.
- Report objectively. (When reporting subjectively, say so.)
- Report the condition of both sides of the body.
- Report calmly and quietly.
- Report as soon after the event as possible so you do not forget details.

General Client Observations

Body Area	Observations
General appearance	Has it changed? If so, in what way? Is there a noticeable odor or smell in the client's room? Does he always complain about the heat or cold?
General mood	Describe the client's actions rather than your interpretation of them. "The client threw a shoe at her daughter" rather than "The client was angry at her daughter." Has it changed? Does he talk a lot or very little? Does he make sense? Can he report things to you accurately? Does he hallucinate (see or hear things)? Is he oriented (knows where he is, who he is, and who you are)? Is he anxious, calm, excited, or worried? Does he talk about pain?

9

Body Area	Observations
General mood (*cont.*)	Does he speak rapidly or slowly? Does he look at you when he speaks? Can he be understood when he speaks? Can he read? Can he remember? Is he confused or forgetful?
Sleeping habits	Have these changed? Is he a quiet or restless sleeper? Does he complain about lack of sleep? Does his report agree with your observations? How many pillows does he sleep with? How much does he sleep?
Pain	Where is the pain? How long does the client say he has had it? Is it new pain? How does he describe it? Is it constant? Does it come and go? Is it sharp, dull, or aching? Has he had medicine for the pain? Does the client say that the medicine relieves the pain? Is there any activity which brings on the pain?
Daily activities	Does the client dress himself? Does the client walk with or without help? What kind of help?
Personal care	Can the client bathe himself? Can the client brush his teeth, comb his hair, go to the bathroom, or wash his face? Does he ask for assistance?
Movements	Does the client limp?
Skeletal system	Pain, limited movement, swelling in joints, warm tender joints, unusual positioning of any body part, redness in joints.
Muscular system	Painful movement, swelling, limited movement, color of skin over painful areas. Does he lie still? Does he change position frequently? What is his favorite position?
Skin	Temperature, texture, moisture, bruises, healing of bruises, incision appearance, mouth condition. Has it changed? Is the client's skin unusually pale (pallor)? Is it flushed (red)? Are his lips or fingernails turning blue (cyanotic)? Is there any swelling (edema) noticeable? Are there reddened or tender areas? Where are they? Is the skin shiny? Is there any puffiness?

10

Body Area	Observations
Circulatory system	Chest pain; swelling of fingers, toes, feet, ankles, around the eyes, pulse rate and quality; color of lips, nails, fingers, toes; headaches; pain in legs when walking.
Respiratory system	Pain while breathing, rate and quality of respirations, cough, sputum (color and consistency), wheezing, shortness of breath, color of fingers and toes.
Digestive system	Pain, appetite, flatus, vomiting (color of vomitus), feces (color, amount, frequency, odor), discomfort before or after eating. Can he control his bowels? Have his eating habits changed? Does he complain he has no appetite? Does he dislike his food? What and how much does he eat? Is he always thirsty? Does he seldom ask for fluids? Is it difficult for him to eat or swallow?
Nervous system	Painful areas of body, twitching, involuntary movement, inability to move, inability to feel stimuli.
Urinary system	Pain during urination; ability to control his urine; urine color, odor, amount, frequency; blood in urine; pain in kidney area.
Eyes	Pain, discharge, redness, sensitivity to light, vision change.
Ears	Pain, discharge, hearing change.
Nose	Pain, discharge, bleeding, smell.
Female genitalia	Menstrual periods (frequency, amount of flow, pain), vaginal discharge (color, odor, amount), breasts (lumps, discharge, soreness, parasites, draining sores).
Male genitalia	Pain, discharge, parasites, draining sores.

TEACHING YOUR CLIENTS

You will teach by example, by discussion, or by taking part in activities with your client. You will often help a client relearn old skills or learn new skills. Everyone learns differently and must have an individualized teaching plan. Adults learn differently than children, and a client with a mental handicap learns differently than one who has had memory loss. Become familiar with each client's individualized teaching plan and follow it closely.

Reasons for Differences in Learning

- Past experiences with learning
- Disease process
- Motivation for learning
- Family dynamics
- General abilities
- Teaching skills of the teacher
- Age

Points to Remember When Teaching a Client

- Be sure the client is paying attention.
- Be sure the client wants to learn.
- Be familiar with the material you are teaching.
- Speak slowly and clearly but not in baby talk.
- Remain calm. Do not lose your patience.
- Do not teach too much at once.
- Teach at times most convenient for the client.
- Leave written materials for the client.

2

Working with People

BASIC HUMAN NEEDS

All people have *basic needs* that must be met so they can survive as human beings. Each need does not have to be met completely each day, but the more needs that are

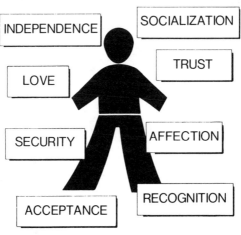

BASIC PSYCHOLOGICAL NEEDS

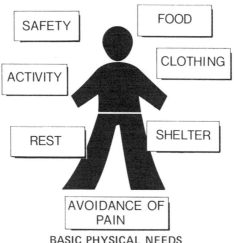

BASIC PHYSICAL NEEDS

met, the better the quality of life. When one need is out of balance due to illness, the other needs are also affected. When a person becomes ill or disabled, it means he is unable to satisfy his needs and your help is needed. Your objective observations of the client and your discussions with your supervisor will help to determine if you are truly meeting the client's needs as stated in the plan of care. If not, changes may be necessary.

PAIN

Pain means different things to different people. A client in pain may

- Have a rapid pulse, shallow and rapid breathing, or show signs of fatigue
- Have increased anxiety and stress
- Withdraw and decrease communication, food, and fluid intake

- Make faces and gestures with their hands, moan, and cry
- Demonstrate angry behavior

To help a client in pain

- Ask what usually decreases his pain. Do not change the routine if it works!
- Talk to the client. Explain your actions before doing them and explain how the client may help.
- Gain the client's confidence.
- Allow the client to move at his own pace. Do not rush him.
- Observe the client for any increase in pain. Alter your care accordingly.
- Report to your supervisor if the client's pain changes or if the medication does not help.

FAMILY

A *family* is a unit bound together by common interests whose members work together to meet the needs of all members. The functions of a family are to

- Protect the members
- Transmit culture
- Meet individual needs
- Maintain stability
- Teach self-sufficiency and survival

Families have changed in the last 35 years. Today

- Families are smaller
- Women go to work
- People live longer
- Society now assumes some of the care of the elderly
- Family members do not always live near one another

- Roles are not carefully prescribed
- The sick can be cared for in institutions

As you enter a family to begin working with one of its members you will become aware of how the family operates. Your responsibility is to work and care for the client within the framework of the family and to help the client live with his illness or disability within this unit. Do not try to change the client or bring in too many new ideas or you may not be welcome. Remember, the client has operated many years within the family unit. When you leave the client's home, he must remain. If you insist that the client change, he may have difficulty with his family.

You may be sent into a home where you are not totally comfortable. These feelings may be due to the family situation or to your own background. Try to review your feelings before you call your supervisor. Are you afraid? Do you understand what is happening in the house? Your supervisor will help you become more comfortable with your feelings and help you understand what is happening. Never leave the client unattended or fail to go to your assignment! If you cannot return to the house, tell your supervisor. Your personal feelings should never keep you from giving the best care you can and leaving the client in a safe manner.

A *role* is the part a person has in his family or in a particular situation. Each family member has a role that has either been learned from older family members or that has been developed over the years. Each person in the family may have several roles. For example, a woman may be a mother, a daughter, and a wife. Each role demands different behavior and has different responsibilities. Balancing these roles is difficult and professional help may be needed.

The *economics* of a family is a very complex issue. Money is spent in each family according to its own rules and beliefs. You may often be asked by one family member to comment on the way another family member spends money. It is important to act in a nonjudgmental manner. You can say, "I'm not really in a position to comment on this situation. I suggest you discuss your feelings directly with the person." If you feel, however, money is being spent in such a way as to injure a family member or cause danger to the family, report your observations to your supervisor immediately.

Family dynamics are the ways in which members of a family function together. *Support systems* include individuals, agencies, and other civic groups that help individuals or families adjust to difficult situations. Sometimes a family can change their family dynamics to meet a crisis; sometimes the adjustment cannot be made without outside help. Be supportive and nonjudgmental as you work to set up a secure and comfortable support system for the family.

Support systems can be formal or informal.

- *Informal system:* people help one another because they want to. This system includes church groups, neighbors, and friends.
- *Formal system:* people help because they are paid to do so, because they have a particular skill or profession, or because an outside agency or the government says they must do so. This system includes the visiting nurse, the homemaker/home health aide, caseworker.
- *Support groups:* people who have similar needs meet together, usually with a leader or facilitator, to discuss and share common problems, help one another, and gain knowledge from one another.

Denial is used by some people when they meet a situation with which they cannot cope. They simply say, "It doesn't exist." This is how they shield themselves from unpleasant situations. The family has the right to deny a situation if that is their method of coping. As the caregiver, you will be asked to deliver the best care within that situation. Keeping in mind the reason the client or the family is denying the truth will help you give better care to the client.

Abusive words and difficult behavior are often used by a client who is angry at a particular situation. A client may focus his anger at you in the form of abusive words, insulting remarks, or threatening behavior. Because you are paid to care for the client he may feel he does not have to be nice to you. He may, however, not be unpleasant to a member of the family, because he is afraid that person may not return to visit him. Another client may be nice to you and not to his family. Still another client may like to make one person jealous to show that he is still in control of the situation.

When you have to deal with difficult behavior, remain calm and try to put the client's actions and words into perspective. Often a client is not aware he is being unpleasant. If you tell him that he is doing or saying something that makes you uncomfortable, he will often stop it. If you have difficulty expressing your feelings, speak to your supervisor. If you feel you are in danger, contact your supervisor immediately.

WORKING WITH CLIENTS WHO ARE ILL OR HAVE A DISABILITY

Each person reacts to illness and being dependent in a different way. Some of the factors affecting both an illness and a disability are:

- Age
- Emotional health
- Diagnosis
- Whether illness or disability is chronic or acute
- Prognosis for recovery or change in condition
- Family
- Economics
- Support mechanisms
- Presence of pain
- Reason for the illness or disability

It is always correct to involve the client in the planning of his care and in the actual care itself. Remember, you will leave, but the client will remain in the home. By establishing a routine in which the client has had a part, you are preparing him to better continue his care when you are gone. Everyone, young and old, regardless of illness or disability, has the right to take part in his care. Clients also have the right to refuse to take part.

As you work with your client

- Promote self-care
- Promote self-respect
- Promote behavior appropriate to the client's condition and age
- Promote a safe, clean environment

MENTAL HEALTH AND MENTAL DISABILITY

Mental health is the ability to function effectively in a certain society. Mental health is the basis for all behavior and relationships with others. Mental health is also a matter of degree. At times everyone shows behavior that may be judged to be unusual. The difference between a mentally healthy person and one with a mental disability is that the person who is mentally disabled adopts characteristics or behavior that no longer enables him to function within society. Mentally healthy people can

- Adapt to change
- Give and receive affection and love
- Tolerate stress to varying degrees
- Accept responsibility for their own feelings and actions
- Distinguish between reality and nonreality
- Form and keep relationships with people

We now know that *mental disabilities* are not contagious and that there are many reasons for these types of disabilities. We also know that some mental disabilities can be cured. A mentally disabled client must be treated with respect. Support him and his family. See to his safety and follow the plan of care.

Some causes of mental disability are

- Isolation
- Medication
- Drugs
- High fevers
- Family and interpersonal relationships
- Environment
- Chronic stress
- Alcohol
- Venereal disease
- Heredity
- Circulatory diseases

Some behaviors which indicate the presence of mental diasability are

- Behavioral changes
- Hallucinations
- Sleeplessness
- Fears
- Decreased memory
- Disorientation
- Forgetfulness
- Mood swings
- Withdrawal

Defense Mechanisms

When a person is subjected to stress, he sometimes reacts defensively. This is normal. When *defense mechanisms* are used so often that a person is not in touch with reality, he is said to be mentally disabled. The most common defense mechanisms include the following:

- *Denial:*   "It is not possible."
- *Depression:*   "It is no use. It is hopeless."
- *Regression:*   Acting like a child or becoming dependent
- *Repression:*   Forgetting about the situation, putting it out of mind
- *Projection:*   "It is not my fault but the fault of the medical people."
- *Rationalization:*   Explaining how one's behavior is acceptable even though it is not
- *Aggression:*   Behavior that attacks everyone regardless of cause

Depression may be an illness, the result of medication, or the defense mechanisms that allow your client to deal with his situation. Some depression is to be expected when your client realizes he does not have as much control over his life as he once did. Signs of depression include

- Lack of interest in activities
- Change in appetite
- Being overly appreciative of help
- Lack of activity or social interaction
- Lack of expression in face or voice

Sometimes a client will remain depressed no matter what you do. Do not become discouraged. Continue to include him in the planning and execution of care. Continue trying to interest him in meaningful activities.

Overdependence can be adopted by a client when he realizes he does not have as much control over his life as he once did. This client then gives up all control and becomes totally dependent on another for his care. Continue to offer this client the opportunity to take part in his care and to take some responsibility. A client will assume his independence when he is ready to meet his own needs. Until that time, it is your responsibility to assume his care.

Caring for the Mentally Disabled

- Provide support for the client's family.
- Encourage your client to take his medication regularly and keep doctors' appointments.
- Report your observations objectively and accurately.
- Maintain a friendly, positive, nonjudgmental manner.
- Encourage your client to take part in his care as appropriate
- Speak to the client in simple sentences. Do not shout or talk baby talk.

SUBSTANCE ABUSE

The term substance abuse refers to the excessive use of drugs or alcohol to the point that behavior is altered. The treatment for substance abuse is not easy and takes a long time. For those individuals who continue treatment the result may be a complete cure. Some misconceptions about substance abuse

- "Everyone does it."
- "I can control it."
- "No one will know."
- "It makes me feel good."

General Signals of Substance Abuse

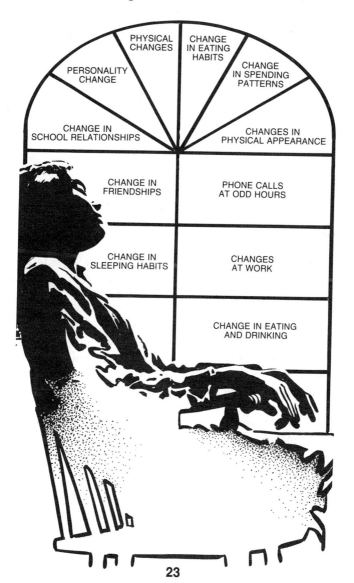

PHYSICAL CHANGES

CHANGE IN EATING HABITS

PERSONALITY CHANGE

CHANGE IN SPENDING PATTERNS

CHANGE IN SCHOOL RELATIONSHIPS

CHANGES IN PHYSICAL APPEARANCE

CHANGE IN FRIENDSHIPS

PHONE CALLS AT ODD HOURS

CHANGE IN SLEEPING HABITS

CHANGES AT WORK

CHANGE IN EATING AND DRINKING

3

Caring for a Geriatric Client

AGING

Geriatrics refers to the knowledge and care of the elderly. If you cannot take care of the elderly because you are afraid or because you have negative feelings about elderly people, tell your supervisor, but do not let these feelings affect your care.

Most elderly people live in their own homes. Some people do not require any assistance to remain independent. Others require daily assistance, while many others can remain independent with assistance only a few times per week.

Each of your clients will age differently. To some it will be just another stage of their life. To others it will be a lonely and frightening time.

Facts of Aging

- The elderly want to remain independent.
- The elderly enjoy sexual relationships.
- The elderly can maintain good health.
- All elderly are not "senile."

- All elderly want to contribute to society and their environment.
- All elderly can learn new tasks although it may take them longer than younger people.

As you care for a geriatric client remember to

- Assist the client as *he* needs it, not as you think he needs it. Let the client take an active part in his care if he wishes to and is able. Observe any changes in his condition.
- Encourage simple, useful activity.
- Provide a safe environment.
- Protect the client from extreme temperatures.
- Provide for warmth and ventilation.
- Teach the client how to maintain his own personal hygiene.
- Dress the client and comb his hair in a style appropriate to his age.
- Speak slowly and in simple sentences. Do not talk baby talk to the client.
- Do not disturb the client's personal belongings or change the placement of furniture unless you discuss it with the client first.
- Always show patience and respect.

Physical Changes of Aging

Body system or organ	Normal aging change	Possible problems or consequences
Skin	Decreased response to pain sensation, temperature changes, and vibration	Accidents, inability to feel hot/cold objects, weather changes, injury, and/or pain

Body system or organ	Normal aging change	Possible problems or consequences
Skin (cont.)	Loss of fat under skin and fatty padding over bony prominences such as hips, change in number of blood vessels	Veins seem prominent, wrinkles appear, especially facial, folds in skin appear, bedsores occur, slower healing, loss of hair
	Decrease number of sweat glands	Difficulty in keeping body temperature constant
	Decrease oil production	Dry skin, itchy, easily injured
	Pigment cells cluster	Moles and "old age spots" (liver spots), graying of hair
Eyes	Clouding of lens	Cataracts
	Decreased ability to focus	Difficulty seeing at night or in fluorescent lighting
	Decreased production of tears	Dry eyes
	Inability to blink quickly	Easier to get a foreign body in the eye
	Muscle degeneration in 50 percent of people over 70	Central vision loss
	Less light reaching retina	Need for good lighting
	Eyelids may evert/invert	Irritation
Ear	Decreased ability to hear high-frequency sounds	Hearing loss
	Stiffness and inflexibility of ear structure	Distortion of sounds, pain if volume is too high

Body system or organ	Normal aging change	Possible problems or consequences
Sense of Taste	Decreased number of taste buds Salty taste decreases the most	Food may become tasteless, excessive use of salt and sugar
Sense of Smell	Declines	Difficulty smelling, smoke, gas, etc., or enjoying pleasant odors
Mouth/Teeth	Loss of gum and bone structure around teeth	Periodontal disease, loss of teeth
Brain	Increased reaction time decline in verbal skills	Slowed reflexes, inability to learn quickly
	Memory loss may occur after age 50	Recall, recognition may be slightly slowed
	Decline of deep sleep	Periods of wakefulness during sleep hours
	Decreased need for sleep	Decrease hours of rest
Lungs/chest	Increased stiffness of respiratory muscles	Decrease in expansion of lungs
	Decreased elasticity of rib cage	Mild barrel chest due to structural changes
	Decreased area for oxygen and carbon dioxide exchange	Decrease of oxygen availability during exercise and rest
	Decreased activity of cilia and diminished cough reflex	Difficulty coughing and eliminating foreign particles from lungs, increase of pneumonia and bronchitis
Heart/ circulatory System	Decreased cardiac muscle strength	Less cardiac output
	Narrowing of arteries	Increased blood pressure

Body system or organ	Normal aging change	Possible problems or consequences
Musculo-skeletal System	Decrease of calcium absorption	Osteoporosis, increased incidence of fractures
	Loss of muscle mass and tone	Fatigue and weakness
Balance	Less efficient balancing mechanism and reactions	Increased incidence of falls, tendency to stand with flexed hips and knees
Gastro-intestinal System	Decreased esophogeal action	Indigestion, slower transport of food to stomach
	Decreased large bowel mobility	Constipation, incomplete emptying of bowel
	Decreased sensitivity to thirst	Dehydration
Renal System	Decreased size of urinary bladder and kidneys, decreased filtration and blood flow to kidneys	Frequency of urination, increased sensitivity to medication, decreased ability to eliminate toxic waste
Genitalia	*Men:* enlarged prostate gland and increased time to urinate	Prostatic obstruction, urinary retention, increase of urinary infections
	Penis may be less hard	Decreased ability to ejaculate
	Women: decreased vaginal and cervical secretions, thinning of vaginal walls	Uncomfortable intercourse, increased time to experience orgasm
	Decreased estrogen after menopause	Increase of male secondary sex characteristics

MENTAL CHANGES

Elderly clients with mental changes must be treated carefully, just as you would treat any impaired client, not as an object of pity or as a child. As you care for the client, do so with patience and understanding. This kind of care takes time. If you feel you are no longer able to care for the client, speak to your supervisor and ask for a change of assignment.

General facts about mental changes are

- Decreased circulation to the brain can cause mental changes.
- Medications can cause mental changes.
- Some social changes can cause mental changes.
- Some mental changes are permanent while others are temporary.
- Not all elderly clients have mental changes.
- People of all ages have mental changes.

Dementia is the gradual decrease of a person's ability to make judgments. This condition is not a normal part of aging and has been called *senility*. *Reversible dementia* is caused by a physical, chemical, or social reason. When the reason is removed, the person usually reverts back to his predementia state. *Irreversible dementia* is usually caused by the loss of small parts of brain tissue due to small strokes, other deteriorating diseases, or Alzheimer's disease.

Discuss your client's behavior with your supervisor. Ask what type of dementia or mental changes your client has so you will understand what causes your client's behavior.

The family of a client suffering from dementia is often stressed.

- Encourage them to seek support from professional groups both for coping and for financial assistance.
- Encourage them to have activities outside of the house.
- Encourage them to "take a break from the care of the client" without feeling guilty.
- Encourage the primary care person to explore the availability of community resources.
- Encourage the family to take an active part in organizations that act on legislation pertinent to the patient's condition.

SOCIAL CHANGES

There are many kinds of social changes

- Retirement
- Change in income
- Change in activity levels
- Isolation from family and friends
- Death of a spouse
- Change in housing
- Increased dependence on others

Some people incorporate these changes into their lives while others become mentally disabled. If you notice changes in your client, report them. Also report any social changes to your supervisor so you can discuss a plan for a possible reaction to the change.

REALITY ORIENTATION

Reality orientation is a technique used to help clients become familiar with their environment on a daily basis. As you use this technique, be sure to remember the following:

- The program must be individualized. Be sure to consult your supervisor *before* it is started.
- The client's family is an important part of the process. If they do not want to take part, discuss this with your supervisor.
- Help the client understand the objects on the board.
- Determine if the client remembers the information and for how long.

REALITY ORIENTATION BOARD

DAY:	Monday
DATE:	Feb 3
YEAR:	1988
WEATHER:	Sunny
ADDRESS:	154 Tulip Street
CITY:	Millville
STATE:	Rhode Island
ACTIVITIES:	•Watch T.V.
	•Clean linen drawer

SPECIAL CONSIDERATIONS IN CARING FOR THE ELDERLY CLIENT

Safety

It is easier to prevent an accident than to heal its consequences. Clients are often unrealistic about their capabilities. Encourage your client to think realistically about his capabilities. You are responsible for protecting the client and those around him. If you are asked to take part in activities that you believe are improper or dangerous, call your supervisor immediately!

- Help provide good lighting with switches that are accessible.
- Encourage the use of grab bars in bathrooms, tub areas, and showers.
- Encourage the use of bannisters.
- Encourage and demonstrate safe practices in the kitchen such as wearing clothes that are not long and flowing; using pot holders; turning pot handles in so they will not be a danger, watching cooking pots so they do not burn, bubble over, or catch fire.
- Set the thermostat on water heaters so that the hot water is at a safe level.
- Be sure smoke detectors are in the house, are properly placed, and are in working order.
- Plan emergency exits from the house.
- Encourage clients to discuss their driving capabilities realistically with their physician.
- Do not permit your client to smoke in bed unsupervised.

Exercise

Planned exercise that is done as part of an overall health plan, reviewed by a physician, is beneficial for all older clients. Benefits from exercise are many.

- Feelings of well-being
- Increased strength to bones
- Increased cardiac and respiratory capacity
- Decreased weight
- Decreased blood pressure
- Decreased anxiety
- Better sleep habits

Medication

Help your client maintain a foolproof, organized method for taking medication. This method should be established by your supervisor with input from you and the client. Be sure all the medications are prescribed for your client and that he is not borrowing a friend's medication. Be aware of the side effects of all of the medication your client takes. Report any reaction to medication or any change in your client. Encourage your client to take all medication to the doctor's office so the physician can review what the client is taking. Help the client throw out old, outdated medication that is no longer used.

Additional facts regarding medication are

- Elderly clients often react to medication differently than younger people.
- The older body uses medication at a different rate than a younger body.
- The kidneys and liver of an older body remove waste products at different rates than in a younger body.
- Elderly clients often forget to take medication or forget that they have taken it and repeat the doses.
- Elderly clients often have several doctors, each of whom is not aware of all the medication that may have been prescribed by other physicians.

Sexuality

Sexual desire does not disappear when people age. Your client may have to change the ways he expresses sexuality due to physical limitations, but all clients should be encouraged and assisted in fulfilling this need. Clients may want the closeness of touching and being held, or other aspects of the sexual act. Clients may have sexual practices that are unfamiliar to you. Discuss these practices with your supervisor if you need any explanation or if you are uncomfortable. Be sure that your feelings concerning sexual activity between older people do not interfere in your relationship with your client. If you are caring for a couple, respect their privacy and confidentiality.

Elderly Abuse

When working in your client's house be aware of any sign of abuse. Abuse can be found in all kinds of homes, in all kinds of economic situations, and in various forms. Be alert! Should you suspect that your client or any member in the house is being abused, report your suspicions to your supervisor immediately!

Signs of Abuse

- Bruises on a client that are hard to explain
- Client demonstrating fear of one person
- Request from a client not to be left alone with a particular person
- Conflicting stories from family members
- A "feeling" that something is not right
- Lack of nourishment for the client
- Lack of family concern for the safety of the client
- Exchange of abusive words between family members
- Unexpected deterioration of the client's health

4

Working with Children

BASIC NEEDS OF CHILDREN

Children are not little adults. They must successfully meet specific needs at a certain age before they can mature. Often when a child is ill or a family member is ill, meeting these needs is difficult. This is your role: to meet the needs of the child.

You may care for a child because the main caregiver

- Becomes ill or suffers a disability
- Needs a rest or assistance with the care
- Must be taught, by your example, how to care for the child
- Must leave the house to work
- Has been reported or suspected of child abuse or neglect

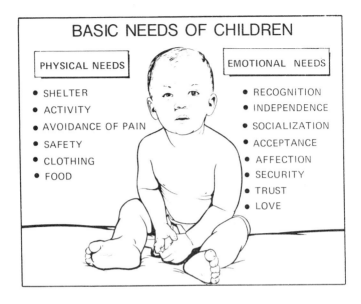

BASIC NEEDS OF CHILDREN

PHYSICAL NEEDS	EMOTIONAL NEEDS

Physical Needs:
- SHELTER
- ACTIVITY
- AVOIDANCE OF PAIN
- SAFETY
- CLOTHING
- FOOD

Emotional Needs:
- RECOGNITION
- INDEPENDENCE
- SOCIALIZATION
- ACCEPTANCE
- AFFECTION
- SECURITY
- TRUST
- LOVE

Stages of Development—Birth to Adolescence

Stage	Key Characteristics or Tasks	Guidelines for Activities
Infancy: Birth to 1 yr	Rapid growth, totally dependent on adults; experiences first relationships; starts to know the world through senses	Provide calm routine within the infant's schedule; encourage stimulation with brightly colored objects tied to crib, music, shapes and textures, swings, carriages, toys that can be put into larger containers

Stage	Key Characteristics or Tasks	Guidelines for Activities
Training period: 1-3 yrs	Begins independence and exploration; learns to say no; puts everything in mouth; shows food preferences; frightened of loud noises; can understand simple honest explanation; may not share; usually starts to toilet train	Attachment to mother and regular caretakers is strong; repeats familiar stories; does not know fact from fiction; help gain familiarity with objects that are part of his care, help toilet train as family wishes with positive reinforcement; likes pull toys, balls, mirrors, threads beads, stackable objects
Love Triangle: 3-5 yrs	Girls mature more quickly; discover sharing of friends and parents; affection and jealousy apparent; imitates; attempts to please; assumes some of own personal care; vivid imagination leads to stories; likes to refuse familiar objects.	Approval of family important; older children like to take part in care; enjoys activities with hands and crayons, easy puzzles, and ball games. Always give simple reasons for activities.
Middle Childhood: 6-12 yrs	Peer acceptance important; easily embarrassed; asserts independence; makes friendships; secretive; argues with adults; growth spurt from 10-12 yrs old; sexual curiosity	Reasons for actions important; explain; give time frame for schedule; enjoys scientific play, jigsaw puzzles, table games, electronic games, music, puppets, crafts, and models

Stage	Key Characteristics or Tasks	Guidelines for Activities
Adolescence: 13-18 yrs	Rapid growth physically and emotionally; sexual development; mood changes; relationships very sensitive; need for privacy; peer relationships and independence very important; suggestions from parents may be rejected but accepted from strangers; concern for appearance.	Respect need for privacy, sexual concerns; explain all actions logically and honestly; enjoys reading, use of telephone, music; encourage expression of ideas and desires.

CHILDREN WITH HANDICAPS

Congenital anomalies (birth defects) are abnormal conditions present at birth that may or may not be noted at that time. Some anomalies are visible such as a hand with only three fingers on it; other anomalies are not visible, such as a child born with only one kidney. Causes for these occurrences range from genetic disorders to exposure to toxic chemicals such as alcohol or drugs.

When you care for a child with an anomaly, you will assist with both the physical care and the emotional acceptance of the situation. It is not unusual for the family to experience guilt, depression, fear, and other emotional difficulties. Show them an accepting behavior and encourage them to discuss their feelings. If you experience certain unfamiliar feelings, discuss them with your supervisor so that you will better understand them.

CHILDREN UNDER STRESS

Children react to stress differently than adults do. As you notice changes in the child's behavior, even if they are small ones, report them to your supervisor so that the plan of care can be modified.

Possible changes in the home are

- Noise restrictions
- Attention restrictions
- Financial changes
- Discussions of family's fear
- Change in their routine
- Change in the mood of child's usual caretaker
- Different caretaker
- Strangers in the house

A change in a child's behavior is the first sign that they are experiencing stress. You may notice

- Refusal to follow familiar household routines
- Shyness, fear, withdrawal
- Jealousy
- Nightmares and fears
- Denial of the condition
- Overdependence
- Bed wetting

DISCIPLINE AND PUNISHMENT

Discipline is a set of rules that governs conduct and actions and results in orderly behavior. *Punishment* is a harsh response to an offense or wrong doing, as when a rule is broken. It is important for you to maintain the discipline in the house. If you have to set up new rules, be sure the client and the family will be able to live with them when you are gone. If you are unable to follow the discipline in the house, or if you think it is the wrong type of discipline, or if you think somebody is in danger, discuss the situation with your supervisor immediately. Punishment is *not* within your role as a home-maker/home health aide.

As you work with children

- Treat each child as an individual.
- Encourage and praise children.
- Use positive suggestions; avoid saying "Don't."
- Make mealtime a pleasure.
- Prepare food the child enjoys.
- Encourage parents to take an active part in decision making.
- Do not take sides in an argument.
- Report changes in family members.
- Report changes in family activities.
- Report feelings or suggestions and the objective happenings which led to your suspicions.
- Report child abuse or neglect.

CHILD ABUSE

Abuse is any act considered to be improper and usually one that causes harm or pain to another. Abuse is found in all types of homes, in all types of cities and towns, and at various ages. Abuse is known to happen in families that are very wealthy and those that are very poor.

It is possible you will be assigned to a client where abuse is taking place and no one knows about the abusive situation. In such a case, you will find out about the abuse by accident. Report it immediately! In some states it is a crime *not* to report such information.

Some Reasons for Abuse

- The abuser was also abused and learned this type of behavior.
- The abuser cannot cope with the stress of having children.
- The abuser is not the parent, but the parent is not able to stop the event.

Reasons Children Do Not Report Abuse

- They are ashamed.
- They do not know whom to tell.
- They do not know any other type of behavior.
- They are afraid the abuse will increase.
- They feel they deserve it.

There are three main kinds of abuse:

Physical: Physical abuse is beating, tying up, or burning. The evidence of this abuse is visible except in the case of broken bones which must be verified by x-ray.

Emotional: Emotional abuse is evident when a child is scared, neglected, screamed at, or permitted to feel unsafe.

Sexual: Sexual abuse occurs when a child is forced to submit to sexual acts because of fear of either physical or emotional harm.

Your Feelings About Child Abuse

Many people have definite feelings about child abuse and the punishment they feel the abusers deserve. Once abuse has been reported and the protection system of the area has taken charge, your role is to work with the system. When you are asked to work in a home where there has been some type of abuse, you will be asked to perform your job without being judgmental or punishing the parents. If you feel you are unable to do this, report your feelings to your supervisor.

When you receive your assignment, be clear about your role, what you are to do and what you are not to do. You will be asked to provide a safe environment for the child and support the parent in learning to cope with the situation and the child. Learning new behavior is very difficult and your support is crucial.

No matter what the case, if you are in a home where child abuse has taken place, here are some general guidelines.

- Be supportive to the parents. Do not be judgmental. Do not compare one case with another. Do not compare their life with yours. We are all different and cope in different ways.
- Be observant! Observe family dynamics. How do the people in the family interact? Do they scream? Do they tease? Do they talk nicely to one member and in a hostile tone to another?
- Are there signs of further abuse? Do the children have marks on them? Are they fed? Is there food in the house? Do the children have a place to sleep? Are they clean? Do they laugh? Do they play? Do they seem afraid?
- Have you noticed any unusual behavior?
- Do the parents have activities that can be considered "adult"?
- Is the family keeping counseling appointments?
- Listen to what the children say about their treatment. If you do not understand what they are telling you, report the whole conversation to your supervisor.

If you suspect something is wrong with the family dynamics, report your feelings and the objective observations to your supervisor immediately! Do not wait! Children cannot always protect themselves. They need adults to do it for them.

DEVELOPMENTAL DISABILITIES

A *developmental disability* is any condition that interferes with proper development of a person. The most familiar developmental disabilities are mental retardation, cerebral palsy, or epilepsy. Although these conditions are permanent, with proper care and teaching, these people can live productive and happy lives.

The reason some people are born with developmental disabilities is not known. Some reasons may be

- Deficit in the development of the fetus
- Infection or injury during birth
- Accident during developmental stages of a child
- Heredity

Children who have developmental disabilities have the same needs as other children. When normal children become adults, they are expected to meet most of their own needs themselves. Your client, however, may never be able to do this. Therefore, you or another adult will have to continue to help your client meet his needs throughout life.

Your feelings as you care for your client are important. Do you feel as though you are doing a worthwhile activity? Do you feel as though you are contributing to the family life of your client? Do you feel that your activities are a waste of time? Discuss your feelings with your supervisor so that the two of you can put your activities into perspective.

The plan of your client's care, is determined by what your client can do at the present time and by what is expected of him in the future.

- Encourage independence up to the ability of the client.
- Provide physical and emotional care.
- Provide a safe general environment.
- Provide a safe environment for feeding and ambulation.

Each family reacts differently to having a disabled member. Do not compare one family with another, but accept all family members as they are. Observe the family dynamics. How do the family members interact with each other? With the client? Do they consider him a part of the family or merely an imposition? Are the family members following the care plan when you are not in the home?

Assisting Children with Taking Medications

The family will always take the responsibility for giving the child his medication. Your role is to be sure the child has been given the medication and to observe him for any possible side effects which include the following:

- Rash
- Difficult breathing
- Vomiting
- Diarrhea
- Irritability
- Pain
- Confusion

NEWBORN AND INFANT CARE

Feeding

Most infants are fed about six times a day or every four hours but some will eat less often and some more often. When you receive your assignment, ask how often the child eats and try to stick to the schedule in the house. You may be asked to bring the baby to the mother when it is time for breast feeding or you may be asked to prepare the formula.

Infants' diets vary. Support the family as they learn to follow the diet their doctor has prescribed. Observe the child for acceptance of the diet.

If you notice a great deal of gas, diarrhea, constipation, or crying immediately after eating, report this to your supervisor immediately. Remember, an infant is unable to get help himself. He needs you to report his distress.

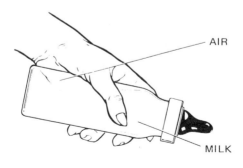

TILT BOTTLE SO
NIPPLE IS ALWAYS
FULL OF MILK

AIR

MILK

CHECK THE
TEMPERATURE OF
THE FORMULA

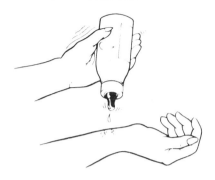

Procedure: Sterilizing Bottles

1. Assemble your equipment: bottles, nipples, caps, jar, bottle brush, dish detergent, hot water from the tap, large pot with cover or special sterilizing pot for baby bottles, small towel, stove, timer or clock, tongs.
2. Wash your hands.
3. Scrub bottles, nipples, and caps with hot soapy water. Use the bottle brush inside the bottles. Squirt hot soapy water through the holes in the nipples to clean out dried-on formula.
4. Rinse bottles, nipples, and caps with hot water.
5. Place a folded small towel in the bottom of the pot. The towel will prevent the bottles from breaking. If you have a rack to hold the bottles, the towel is not necessary.
6. Stand the washed bottles on the towel in a circle or in the rack.
7. Place the caps and the nipples in the clean jar. Place the jar into the pot in the center of the bottles. Place the tongs into the pot so that you can take them out without putting your hand into the water

46

Hold the infant in a safe, comfortable position for feeding and burping.

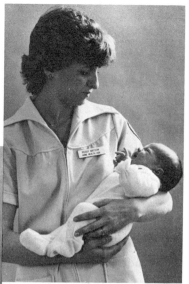

CRADLE POSITION

UPRIGHT POSITION

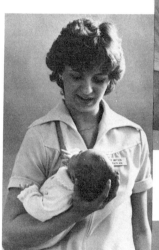

FOOTBALL POSITION

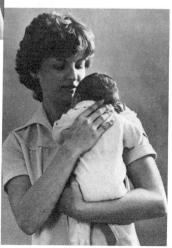

47

8. Pour water into and around the bottles and into the jar with the nipples until 2/3 of each bottle is under water. Cover the pot and place it on the heat source set at the highest setting.

9. After the water comes to a boil, allow the covered pot to boil for 25 minutes. Turn the burner off. Allow the pot to cool.

10. While the pot is cooling, take the tongs out of the water without putting your hand into it. With the tongs, remove the jar of nipples and caps. Stand the jar on a table to cool.

11. Remove the sterile bottles from the pot with the tongs.

12. Empty the water out of the pot. The pot is still sterile, so you can use it for mixing formula.

13. Wash your hands

Ready-to-Use Formula

- Refrigerate only after opening the can.
- Wash the top of the can before opening.
- Shake the can before opening.
- Use a sterilized can opener to open the can.
- Pour the formula into a sterilized bottle and screw on a sterilized cap and nipple.
- Refrigerate all bottles until they are ready for use.

Prefilled Bottles of Ready-to-Use Formula

- Be sure the top of the bottle is clean and dry.
- Unscrew the top and put a sterilized cap and nipple on the bottle.
- Refrigerate the unused portion of the bottle.

Powdered Formula

- Wash and dry all cans before opening.
- Use a sterilized can opener to open the can.
- Follow the directions on the can carefully. They will tell you how much water and how much powder to mix together.

- Be sure to use sterilized water when mixing the formula.
- Be sure all the utensils you use are sterilized.
- Pour the formula into a sterilized bottle and screw on a sterilized cap and nipple.
- Refrigerate all bottles until ready to use.

Concentrated Liquid Formula

- Wash the top of the can before opening.
- Shake the can before opening.
- Use a sterilized can opener to open the can.
- Mix the formula in sterile bottles or a sterile pitcher.
- Refrigerate all mixed formula and all unused concentrate.

Storing Formula

- Formula can be refrigerated up to two days without spoiling. Throw formula away if it is older than two days or if you do not know when it was opened or mixed.
- Mark the opening date on the cans you put in the refrigerator to store.
- Formula starts to spoil within two hours if it is left at room temperature. Keep all bottles refrigerated until 10 minutes before you feed the baby.
- If refrigeration is not available, discuss with your supervisor the best way to store the formula.

Burping

Air in the gastrointestinal tract can cause vomiting and abdominal pain. Prevent this by feeding the baby slowly and burping him after every two ounces of formula. You can burp the baby in one of two ways, as shown in the illustration on the top of page 50.

Observing the Infant's Stool

Observation of the infant's stool or bowel movement is important. A baby is *constipated* when he has difficulty in

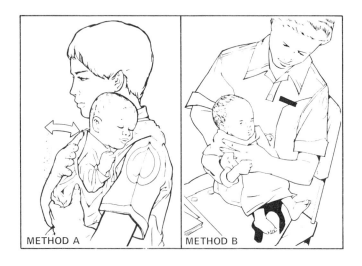

METHOD A

METHOD B

moving his bowels. He has diarrhea when the movements are watery. Diarrhea in infants can be serious and can lead to dehydration. If the stools are watery or green in color or have a foul odor, call your supervisor immediately. Diarrhea can be caused by an allergy or bacteria. To avoid transmitting bacteria to the baby be sure to wash your hands each time you pick him up. Encourage anyone who handles the baby to do the same.

A bottle-fed baby has one to three stools a day which are yellow or mustard in color and lumpy but soft. A breast-fed baby will also have yellow stools but the color may change if the mother eats certain foods. These stools are smoother and looser than those of a bottle fed baby and may occur at every feeding.

Diapers

Every family will chose the type of diapers they will use. There are many brand names and many kinds of diapers available. It is important for you to follow the wishes of the family.

- Change the diapers often to decrease odor and irritation of the baby's skin.
- Clean the baby's genital area each time you change the diaper. Apply powder, lotion, or cream as you have been instructed.
- If you use cloth diapers, rinse the stool from them in the toilet before you put them in the diaper pail.
- If you use rubber pants on top of cloth diapers, be sure the elastic is loose enough to allow air to circulate in the pants.
- Do not use rubber pants over disposable diapers as they already have protection.
- Do not flush disposable diapers down a toilet. Dispose of them as the family wishes and as you know to be aspectically correct.
- Observe the baby's skin each time you change the diaper for change of color, texture, and discharge. Report any changes to your supervisor.

Care of the Umbilical Cord

- Do not give the infant a tub bath until the cord has fallen off.
- Keep the diaper folded away from the cord to decrease the chance of infection and irritation.
- With every diaper change, wash the cord with plain rubbing alcohol on a cotton ball. This speeds up the drying process and decreases infection.
- Never pull the cord off. Let it fall off by itself. Laying the infant on his belly will not hurt him.
- Do not use binders or belly bands.
- Report *any* oozing.

Circumcision

Circumcision is the surgical removal of the loose piece of skin (foreskin) at the end of the penis. This is an elective procedure and must be requested by the parents. Not all male children are circumcised. Sometimes it is done at birth in the operating room. The removal of this skin eliminates the possibility of the foreskin shrinking and thus constricting the penis in later life. Although this does not always occur, when it does, it is very painful. In the Jewish faith, there is a ritual circumcision on the seventh day after birth. This circumcision can be done either at home or in the hospital.

Be sure to follow the physician's instructions after the circumcision. Be sure to ask about bathing the infant.

- Keep the penis protected from rubbing against the diaper.
- Keep the penis clean and free of fecal matter.
- Report any bleeding or drainage.

Bathing

Do not leave the baby alone, even for a minute, while you are bathing him. Do not answer the phone or talk to anybody out of the room. Do not take your eyes off the baby. Keep your hands on the baby at all times.

A *sponge bath* means gently washing each part of the body with mild soap and water but not putting the infant in water. A sponge bath can be done daily and is always done before the umbilical cord has fallen off.

- Clear off a safe place before you sponge the baby.
- Prepare all the equipment before you bring the baby to the area.

- Wash, rinse, and dry one body part at a time.
- Keep the baby covered and warm.

A *tub bath* can be given with the approval of the physician.

Procedure: Giving the Infant a Tub Bath

1. Assemble your equipment: infant tub or sink, two bath towels, cotton balls, washcloth, warm water, baby soap and shampoo, clean clothes, and diaper.
2. Wash your hands and clean the sink or tub.
3. Line the sink with a towel to prevent the baby from slipping.
4. Place a towel nearby to put the baby on after the bath is finished.
5. Fill the tub with 1 to 2 inches of warm water.
6. Undress the baby, wrap him in a towel or blanket and bring to the tub or sink.

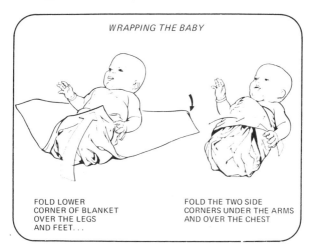

WRAPPING THE BABY

FOLD LOWER CORNER OF BLANKET OVER THE LEGS AND FEET...

FOLD THE TWO SIDE CORNERS UNDER THE ARMS AND OVER THE CHEST

7. Moisten both cotton balls with warm water. Using a separate cotton ball for each eye, gently wipe the infant's eyes from the nose toward his ear.

8. Hold the infant in football style, with the head over the tub. Wet the head with a small amount of water, put a small amount of shampoo on the head, and Rub gently. Rinse well. Dry the head with a towel.

9. Unwrap the infant and put him gently into the water.

10. If the infant is a female, always wash the perineal area from front to back.

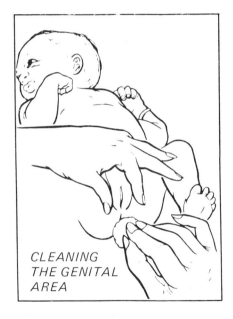

CLEANING
THE GENITAL
AREA

11. If the infant is a boy and uncircumcised, gently pull the foreskin back to clean the penis.

12. After carefully washing and rinsing the infant, wrap him in a towel and dry him thoroughly. You can apply powder or lotion as the mother prefers. Diaper and dress the infant and put him in a safe place.

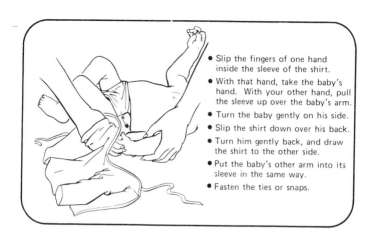

- Slip the fingers of one hand inside the sleeve of the shirt.
- With that hand, take the baby's hand. With your other hand, pull the sleeve up over the baby's arm.
- Turn the baby gently on his side.
- Slip the shirt down over his back.
- Turn him gently back, and draw the shirt to the other side.
- Put the baby's other arm into its sleeve in the same way.
- Fasten the ties or snaps.

13. Clean the tub and sink and wash your hands.

Infant Safety

- Never leave an infant unattended on a bed, counter, or chair.
- Always put the sides up on the crib when you leave.
- Place the baby on his side or belly after feeding to prevent aspiration.
- Keep all medication and cleaning products locked away from the baby's reach.

5

Care of the Dying
in the Home

DYING

You will often care for a client who is dying. You may feel uncomfortable, helpless, sad, or even frightened. You may even be unsure how to act. Use the same caring, consideration, and understanding you use with clients who will recover.

A client is usually told by his physician that he is dying. Occasionally, a family member may tell the client. Sometimes the client will never actually be told, but he will guess he is dying from the activity around him and the fact that his condition is not improving. If a family decides *not* to let your client know he is dying, you are obliged to carry out their wishes even though at times keeping up the charade is most difficult.

STEPS IN DYING

Doctor Elisabeth Kubler-Ross found there are certain stages, or steps, involved in the dying process.

Step 1—*Denial:* "Not me!"

Step 2—*Anger:* "Why me?"

Step 3—*Bargaining:* "Me, but. . ."

Step 4—*Depression:* "Ah, me. . ."

Step 5—*Acceptance:* "Yes, me."

It is most important to remember that

- All clients are different.
- The family of the person who is dying will go through all of these steps.
- Everyone will not experience every step.
- Clients and families will go from step to step at any time.
- Clients do not go through these steps in any given order.

SPECIAL EMOTIONAL NEEDS

Dying clients are still living people and have the same needs as your other clients. They need

- *To be normal,* to know that the thoughts and feelings they have are like those of others in their situation
- *Meaningful relationships,* a chance to talk to friends and family members on a meaningful level
- *Love,* to feel that they are the object of someone's love; couples may have sexual exchanges
- *Recreation,* some way to pass the time, such as knitting, playing cards, watching T.V., or reading
- *Safety,* to know that they will be carefully cared for up until the moment of death

BE A GOOD LISTENER

When a client suspects he is going to die, he may

- Ask everyone about his chances for recovery
- Be afraid to ask a lot of questions
- Seem to complain constantly
- Make requests that seem unreasonable

Usually, when a client asks questions he is sending a signal that he wants information. You may not have all the information needed to answer the questions. Assure the client that you will either get the information or provide someone who will.

- *Be honest.* If you do not know the answer, say so.
- *Do not offer false hope or reassurance.* Offer short-term realistic goals or say nothing.
- *Do not say too much.* A caring look, an unhurried manner, a nod or word at the right time tells the client you care.
- *Let the client take the lead.* Often a question represents a fear or concern. He may feel relieved if you allow him to express the concern.
- *Do not destroy hope.* If the client really feels he will recover, do not destroy his hope. The client who has hope usually lives longer than the one who does not.

HOSPICE

Many areas of the country have *hospice* programs. These are organized systems of professional care that help families care for dying clients at home up to and including the time of death. Hospice is not appropriate for everyone because not everyone is able to die at home without any heroic measures. Most hospice clients do not wish any treatment except to remain comfortable and pain free. This concept may be difficult for some families to accept.

Hospice

- Treats the client and his family as one unit of care
- Allows the client and family as much choice as possible in determining care in the home
- Makes use of a team of professionals who are experienced in home health care and in care of the dying
- Helps the family through the dying process
- Helps the family after the death of their loved one

PHYSICAL CARE OF THE DYING

Skin care. Bathe daily, with partial bathing as necessary. The skin may be fragile, so wash gently with mild soap. Apply lotion to bony prominences.

Positioning. Do not use tight clothing, stockings, garters, or tight bed linens. Use pillows and rolled blankets for careful positioning. Change the client's position at least every 2 hours. Change soiled linens and protective pads. Change nonsterile dressings when soiled. Reinforce sterile dressings.

Mouth care. Cleanse teeth and mouth at least twice daily. Remove dentures or brush teeth. Cleanse mucus membranes with glycerine swabs as needed.

Bowel care. Keep a careful record of bowel movements and notify the nurse if the client has not had a bowel movement in several days.

Circulation. The circulation slows as death approaches and the arms and legs may feel cold and look ashen. Elevate the limbs as needed to aid blood return. Do not allow the limbs to be in a dependent position.

Food/Water. Assist the client to a comfortable position, cleanse his mouth. Wash his hands, refresh the linen. Air the room of any odors. Do not try to mask odors with perfume or spray, but remove the source of the odors. Ask the client and his family about food choices and try to get as much variety as possible. Offer small portions of food and frequent sips of water so as not to tire the client with long meals. Arrange portions in a neat, appetizing manner.

Breathing. Remove secretions from the mouth. Urge the client to "cough up" mucus. To ease breathing, elevate the head of the bed or prop up the client on pillows.

The Moment of Death

Dying is a spiritual process for some people. Many clients will ask to see a priest, minister, or rabbi. As the time of death nears, services or prayer rituals may be held at the bedside. Respect the family's privacy at this time.

It is very difficult to predict anyone's behavior at the exact moment of death. Some people simply slip into a coma for days before death, and others will cling constantly to a loved one's hand.

Sometimes before death breathing becomes very irregular and may even stop for periods of up to 30 seconds. This is called *Cheyne-Stokes breathing* and is a very usual occurrence. As death approaches, the gurgling breathing called the *death rattle* may begin. At this time the client is usually unconscious. Talk openly and in a concerned way even though it appears the client does not hear you. Hearing is the last sense to be lost and loving words from a family member, up until the moment of death, are comforting.

Plan with your supervisor exactly what you will do when death occurs. It is important to know whom you will call, what you will do, and what your role will be with the grieving family. Be sure you have the telephone numbers of the appropriate people.

Your reaction to the actual death depends on your experience with death, your culture, your religion, and your relationship with the client and his family. Usually, you will feel sadness and a loss when a client dies. If you do not feel a discussion with your supervisor is enough, ask for assistance and support with your feelings.

POSTMORTEM CARE

Care of the body after death is called *postmortem care.* Most of the time, when death occurs at home, the family has been prepared for what to do by the doctor and nurse who care for the client. Usually the client's doctor, the nurse from the home health agency, and the funeral director are notified. If the client's doctor is not available to make a home visit, and the state does not permit the nurse to pronounce the client, an ambulance may have to be called to take the client to the local emergency room so a physician can pronounce him. Check with your agency for the policies and procedures to follow at the time of death.

After death occurs, the family may sit at the bedside and say their final goodbyes. Families handle grief in many ways, and they should have time and privacy as needed. Be sure to inquire about specific religious practices that should be observed at this time.

When appropriate, prepare the body in the following manner:

- Remove all pillows, except under the head.
- Bathe the body, removing secretions, reinforce dressings.
- Place dentures in the mouth, if possible.
- Close the eyes, but do not press on the eyeballs.
- Keep the body flat on its back, straightening the arms and legs.
- Move the body gently to avoid bruising.
- Check with the family regarding any jewelry the client may be wearing.
- Check your agency's policy about removal of catheters. Usually you will not be asked to remove a tube after death if you did not care for it when the client was alive.

After the body is removed from the home, strip the bed and air the room. Remove any equipment. Check with the family regarding the proper disposal of these items. Place personal items carefully at the bedside so family members can remove them at the appropriate time.

In addition, you may help the family by answering phone calls from friends and neighbors, making coffee, or sitting with grieving family members. Ask the family how you can help and try to do whatever is necessary to help them through this difficult time.

6

Infection Control in the Home

MEDICAL ASEPSIS IN THE HOME

It is known that some diseases are caused by *microorganisms*. Although some microorganisms are helpful to people, others cause disease and infection and are called *pathogens*. Pathogens destroy human tissue with their waste products called *toxins*, which are poisonous to the human body.

**Microorganisms
are Everywhere**

- In the air we breathe
- On our bodies
- In our clothing
- In liquids
- In food
- On animals
- In animals
- In human waste
- In animal waste

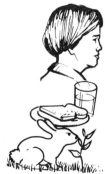

Ways that Microrganisms Are Spread

- Touching secretions, urine, feces
- Touching objects:
  Dishes
  Bed linen
  Clothing
  Instruments
  Belongings
- Sneezing
  Coughing
  Talking
- Contaminated:
  Food
  Drugs
  Water or blood
- Dust particles and moisture in the air

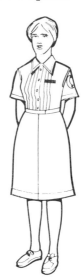

Conditions Necessary for Microorganisms to Grow

- Moisture
- Temperature
- Oxygen
- Darkness
- Nourishment

Medical asepsis means preventing the conditions that allow pathogens to live, multiply, and spread. You will share the responsibility for preventing the spread of disease by using aseptic technique. Reasons for medical asepsis are

- Helping the client overcome a current infection or preventing the spread of that infection

- Protecting the client against *reinfection* or becoming infected a second time by the same microorganism
- Protecting the client against *cross-infection* or becoming infected by a new or different type of microorganism
- Protecting the family and health team against becoming infected by microorganisms passed from caregiver to client or from client to caregiver. Diseases that can be passed from one person to another are called *communicable diseases*.
- Protecting the client from *self-inoculation* or becoming infected with his own organisms

Clean and Dirty Areas in the House

One way to control the spread of disease is to have a clean area and a dirty area in the house.

Clean means uncontaminated and refers to those articles and places from which disease cannot be spread. Clean areas contain food, dishes, and clean equipment. No waste material is ever brought into these areas.

Dirty refers to those areas and articles that have come in contact with disease-causing or carrying agents. In the home, there are degrees of dirty. There is a difference between being dirty with human waste, such as wound drainage or fecal matter, and bed sheets that are only soiled. Articles that are dirty with potentially infectious material are brought into the dirty area for initial cleaning or disposal. Articles that are only soiled are cleaned in the usual way.

HANDWASHING

Washing your hands is the best way to prevent the transfer of microorganisms from one person to another and from an object to a person. Wash your hands frequently!

- Handwashing must be done before and after each task and before and after direct client contact.
- The water faucet is always considered dirty. Use a paper towel to turn the faucet on and off.
- If your hands accidentally touch the inside of the sink, do the whole procedure again.
- Take soap from a dispense, rather than use a bar of soap. The bar of soap leaves pools of soapy water in the soap dish and is considered contaminated.
- Handwashing is effective only when you
  —use enough soap to produce lots of lather
  —rub skin against skin to create friction
  —rub your hands two minutes with soap
  —rinse from the clean to the dirty parts of your hands
  —rinse with running water from two inches above the wrists to the fingertips

Procedure: Handwashing

1. Assemble your equipment: soap or detergent, paper towels, warm running water (if possible), wastepaper basket, nail brush.
2. Open a paper towel near the sink for your clean area. Put all your equipment on it. Leave it there until you are ready to leave the house.
3. Turn the faucet on with a paper towel held between your hands and the faucet. Discard the paper towel in the wastepaper basket.
4. Completely wet your hands and wrists under the running water. Keep your fingers pointed downward. Hold your hands lower than your elbows while washing.
5. Apply soap or detergent to your hands. Work up a good lather over the entire area of your hands and wrists. Get soap under your nails and between your fingers. Use a nail brush on your nails.

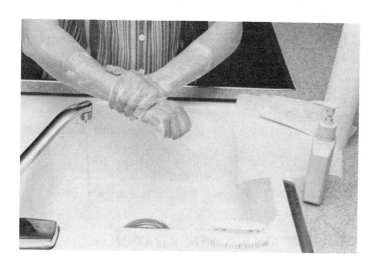

6. Wash with a rotating and rubbing (friction) motion for one full minute.
   a. Rub vigorously.
   b. Rub one hand against the other hand and wrist.
   c. Rub between your fingers by interlacing them.

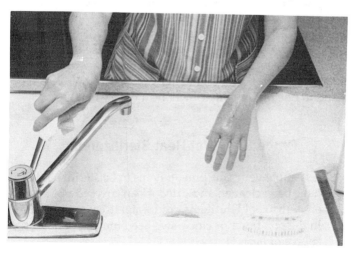

   d. Rub up and down to reach all skin surfaces on your hands and between your fingers.

   e. Rub the tips of your fingers against the palms to clean with friction around the nail beds.

7. Wash at least two inches above your wrists.

8. Rinse well one hand at a time. Rinse your hands. Hold hands and fingertips pointed downward under the water.

9. Dry your hands thoroughly with paper towels.

10. Use a paper towel to turn off the faucet.

11. Throw the paper towel into the wastepaper basket.

DISINFECTION AND STERILIZATION

Disinfection is the process of destroying as many harmful organisms as possible and slowing down the growth and activity of the organisms that cannot be destroyed. *Sterilization* is the process of killing all microorganisms including spores. *Spores* are bacteria that form hard shells around themselves as a defense. Spores are very difficult to kill. Some can live even in boiling water.

Sterilization of equipment is necessary if the article comes in contact with a wound, as in the case of surgical instruments or solutions used for cleaning wounds. In the home, depending on the item, an article can be sterilized in one of two ways—wet heat or dry heat.

Procedure: Wet Heat Sterilization

1. Assemble your equipment: items to be sterilized that have been cleaned and dried, clean covered pot large enough to hold the items, cold water to cover the items in the pot, timer or clock, sterilized tongs, pot holder, source of heat.

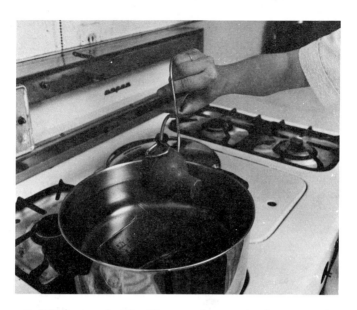

2. Wash your hands. Place equipment in the pot so the water touches all parts of it. Put a clean piece of cloth in the bottom of the pot to protect any glass parts.

3. Cover the contents with cold water. Be sure there is "head room" left in the pot.

4. Put the pot on the source of heat. Bring the contents to a boil. Do not open the pot. Note the steam escaping from under the top. Boil undisturbed for 20 minutes.

5. Turn off the heat. Allow the contents to cool undisturbed. Leave the equipment in the pot until you are ready to use it.

6. Remove the contents with sterilized tongs to a sterilized holder.

Procedure: Dry Heat Sterilization

1. Assemble your equipment: pie tin, dressing or cloth to be sterilized, oven, pot holder.

2. Wash your hands.
3. Place the clean dressing wrapped in a clean cloth into the pie tin.
4. Place the pie tin into an oven heated to 350 degrees. Allow the dressing to bake for one hour.
5. Allow the dressing to cool.
6. Unwrap carefully. Do not touch the dressing as it is considered sterile.

Note: A hot iron held on a dressing for several seconds also sterilizes. However, the oven method is preferred.

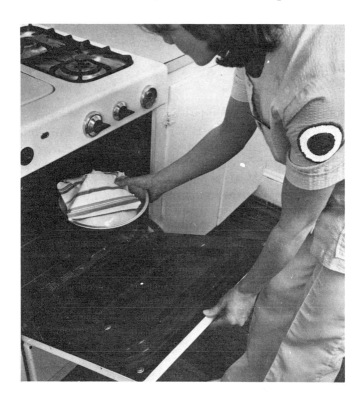

SPECIAL INFECTION CONTROL PRECAUTIONS FOR TRANSMITTABLE DISEASES

Several diseases which are now cared for in the home require the practice of special precautions to lower the chance of transmission from the client to the caregiver. Two of these diseases are AIDS and hepatitis B. You may have feelings about the people who have these diseases because some may have a very different life style from yours. If you do not know the facts about the disease, you may also be afraid. Discuss these feelings with your supervisor, but do not let them get in the way of giving your client the best possible care.

Each agency has its own policies and procedures when caring for clients with these diseases. Ask what policies your agency has. Here are some basic rules:

Sharp objects, needles, blades. Handle these items carefully to prevent cutting yourself. These objects should be placed in a container that is puncture resistant and disposed of according to local rules. Do not bend needles or try to recap them.

Exposure to body fluids or blood. Wear gloves if a chance exists for contamination. If splattering is possible, wear a gown and mask. Flush these waste products down the toilet. Spills should be wiped up by a person wearing disposable gloves using soap and water. The area then should be wiped down with a solution of one part household bleach and ten parts water. The rag should be thrown out in a double plastic trash bag, and the dirty water flushed down the toilet.

Dressings. Wrap these items in a double plastic bag and dispose of them according to local laws.

Plates, glasses, dishes. Use separate disposable utensils if possible. Clean reusable utensils in hot water and detergent following use. Rinse with bleach solution, then rinse with hot water again.

Laundry. Unsoiled laundry should be washed or dry cleaned normally. Soiled linen should be kept separated and handled with disposable gloves. Keep soiled linen in a double plastic bag lined with a cloth bag or pillow-case. Wash linen in machine by emptying contents of plastic bag without touching the items. Throw away the plastic bag. Wash soiled linen each day.

- *Machine washing* (colorfast)

  Use: one cup household bleach in hot water and laundry detergent.

- *Handwashing* (colorfast)

  Use: two tablespoons household bleach in one gallon warm water and laundry detergent

- *Machine washing* (noncolorfast)

  Use: one cup Lysol in warm water and laundry detergent. Rinse well.

- *Hand washing* (noncolorfast)

  Use: two tablespoons Lysol in one gallon warm water and laundry detergent. Rinse well.

7

Care of the Client's Environment

HOMEMAKING

Your housekeeping assignments are based upon the professional assessment of the needs in the home and are related to client care. If the client and his family do not understand your assignment or think you should do more, let your supervisor know.

- Clean environments keep harmful bacteria under control and decrease the spread of communicable diseases.
- Accidents are prevented in areas that are kept orderly, especially the stairs and entrance ways.
- Clean environments contribute to a sense of well-being.

Cleaning a Client's Home

Clean usually refers to an area that is free of pathogens and of clutter. Find out what is clean to your client. Try to meet the client's values. If your values and the client's needs are very different, consult your supervisor.

- If there are many housekeeping tasks to do, discuss them with all family members. Encourage all family members to become part of the plan of action.
- Agree who will do the jobs and when they will be done. Develop a routine.
- If someone is willing to help but does not know how, offer to teach him.

Supplies are necessary to keep a house clean. Try to use the products that are already in the house.

Necessary Supplies	*Nice to Have*
Hot water	Dustpan
Soap or detergent	Vacuum cleaner
Broom	Scouring pad
Vinegar	Mop
Scrub pad, scrub brush	Wastebaskets
Baking soda	
Baking powder	
Pail	
Trash container	

Basic Kinds of Cleaning Products

Products	Uses	Form	Cautions
Soaps and detergents	All types of cleaning; personal cleaning	Liquid, powder, solid	Read labels; protect eyes
All-purpose cleaner	All types of cleaning	Liquid, powder, solid	Read labels; protect eyes
Abrasives/ bleach	Surface soil; kills some pathogens	Liquid, powder	Read labels; protect eyes and skin
Specialty	Specific jobs; windows, metals, etc.	Foam, liquid, powder, spray	Read label

Using Common Cleaning Products

Task	Product	Use
Bathtub stain	White vinegar or paste of hydrogen peroxide and baking powder	Rub stain with rag dipped in vinegar; rinse; leave paste on stain overnight; rinse
Tile cleaner	Sprinkle baking soda	Rub with damp rag; rinse as this makes tiles slippery
Windows and painted surfaces	Mix carefully: 5 cups water; 1 tsp. detergent; 1 pt. rubbing alcohol; ½ cup sudsy ammonia	Wash area carefully; rinse well; dry
Mattress stain	Mix carefully: ½ cup water; ½ cup white vinegar; 1 tsp. detergent	Dab solution on stain; let dry; rub area with water and detergent; leave on for 10 minutes; blot dry; rinse; let dry

Dusting

- Use a rag of lint-free material.
- Dampen the rag with a light spray of water or commercial spray to keep the dust from spreading.
- Dust with motions that will gather the dust, not spread it.

Washing Dishes

- Place dishes on the counter in the order they are to be washed, that is, least dirty first.
- When water is not plentiful, use a dishpan in which you wash the dishes instead of letting the water run as you wash.
- Drain dishes on drainboard.
- Dishes are more sanitary if allowed to air dry.

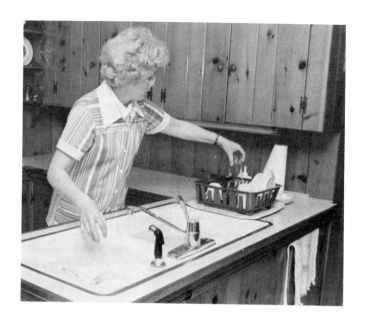

Cleaning the Kitchen

- Wipe up food spills and grease as they occur.
- Keep the refrigerator clean. Do not use sharp objects to scrape off ice or dried-on food. If the refrigerator needs defrosting, discuss this with your supervisor.

Cleaning the Bathroom

- Keep floors dry.
- Maintain good safety in the bathroom. Use nonskid rugs, grab bars, good lighting, and good ventilation.
- Clean the toilet when it is necessary. Do not use the rag for anything else. Wash the rag well after this task.
  —Lift the seat and put soap, detergent, or toilet cleanser into the bowl.
  —Using a toilet brush, scrub the inside of the toilet.
  —Do not mix the toilet cleanser with anything else.

—Be sure to rinse the cleanser from the toilet.

—If there are rust stains, let the cleanser stand in the bowl before you scrub it.

Care of Rugs and Carpeting and Floors

Remove scatter rugs or tack them down so they are not a hazard. Frequent vacuuming or sweeping will preserve the rugs and decrease the lint and dust in the house. Use the vacuum at a time when it will not disturb the family. Ask how to change the "dirt bag." If you find a stain and the family says it is a new one, try to get it out by using a commercial stain remover or mixing baking soda and water into a solution, rubbing it onto the stain, and allowing it to dry. Then vacuum the area.

Cleaning the Floors

- Sweep floors frequently, especially before washing them.
- Wood floors often require special cleaners. Do not use water.
- Do not let water remain on any floor.
- Most households have a mop they use to wash the floor. If you do not find it, discuss this with your supervisor.
- After washing let the floor dry before walking on it or putting furniture back into place.

Pests and Bugs

Pests and bugs may carry disease and can be annoying to you and your client. They may bite, cause skin irritations, or even frighten people. The best way to keep an area free of bugs or rodents is to keep it clean and free of clutter. If you or any member of the family wish to use a commercial product to get rid of bugs or pests, ask your supervisor to be sure it is safe.

- Put food away in closed containers. Clean up spills and crumbs.
- Keep the garbage and trash outside in closed containers.
- Roaches and mice can pass through small cracks in walls and near pipes. Talk to your supervisor about having someone caulk up such holes.
- Do not let water stand inside the house or out of doors.

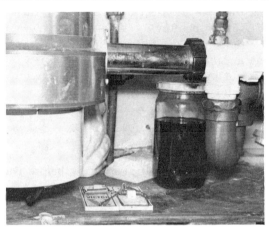

Doing A Client's Laundry

Check all clothes for tears, loose buttons, or frayed edges before washing them. Repair them before washing. Sort clothes by

> *Color.* Dark colors should be washed separately from light colors.
>
> *Fabric.* Delicate fabrics cannot take as much scrubbing as heavy-duty fabrics.
>
> *Degree of dirt.* Wash heavily soiled items together. Heavily soiled clothes should not be washed with those that are only lightly soiled.

If you have any questions about the washing machine, ask the client or a family member. If you use the dryer, take the clothes out immediately so that they will need less ironing. Drying clothes out of doors conserves energy and gives the clothes a fresh smell.

Some homes do not have washing machines. After you have found out how the laundry is usually done in the home, discuss with your supervisor what your responsibilities will be. Bending and lifting wet, heavy laundry could cause you to injure your back. If you must do this, however, use good body mechanics. Protect your back.

Bedmaking

People have various types of sleeping arrangements. A client may sleep in a hospital bed in a separate room from the rest of the family. A client may sleep on the couch. A client may sleep in his own bed. It is your responsibility to keep the bed free of food particles and free of wrinkles. Sometimes your client will need side rails to protect him from falling out of bed and to help him change position while in bed. Side rails can be bought, rented, or improvised.

When you make an occupied bed, ask the client if he prefers the pillow to remain under his head as you work. Keep the client covered and warm and safe as you change the linen. This is especially important since most occupied beds are changed following a bed bath. Talk to your client as you work and tell him what you are doing. Observe him. If he should need your attention, stop the procedure and meet the client's needs immediately.

- Use linen the client has available. If you do not have enough, report to your supervisor.

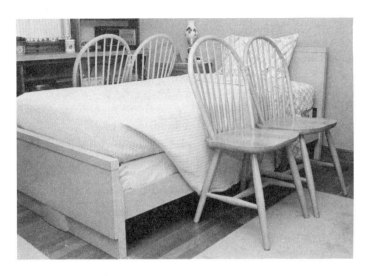

- Try to make the bed according to the custom of the house. If you must make a change, explain your reasons to the client and the family.
- Do not use a torn piece of linen. It may tear more and be dangerous.
- Never use a pin on any item of linen.
- Do not shake the bed linen. Shaking spreads harmful microorganisms to everything in the room and to your uniform.
- Never allow linen to touch your uniform.
- Never put dirty linen on the floor. Put it in a place agreed upon by the family.
- When draw sheets are not available, use a large sheet folded in half widthwise. The fold must always be placed toward the head of the bed and the hems toward the foot of the bed. You can also use a tablecloth for a drawsheet.
- If you must protect the bed, and do not have a plastic bed protector or draw sheet, a plastic tablecloth is excellent. The plastic should never touch the skin.

Always cover it with a cotton draw sheet. Never use plastic from a garment bag or a garbage bag.

- To save linen and washing, use a used clean top sheet as a draw sheet or bottom sheet.
- If your client does not use the bed a great deal, the linen may not have to be changed every day. Evaluate the situation each day.
- Always use good body mechanics when you are making a bed.
- To save time and energy, make one side of the bed first, then move to the other side and complete the job.

Procedure: Making an Occupied Bed

1. Assemble equipment near the bed in the order of its use: two large sheets, a plastic draw sheet, a cotton draw sheet, a disposable bed protector, one bath blanket if available, one bedspread, and a container for dirty laundry.
2. Wash your hands.
3. If you are working on a hospital bed, lower the backrest and knee rest to the flat position. Raise the bed to its highest position.
4. Loosen all the sheets around the bed.
5. Raise the side rail on the opposite side from where you will be working.
6. Take the bedspread and blanket off the bed and fold them neatly.
7. Cover the client with the bath blanket. Ask the client to hold it in place. If he is unable to do this, tuck the edges of the bath blanket under his shoulders. Without exposing him, pull the top sheet off under the bath blanket. If you will use this sheet again, fold it neatly.
8. If the mattress has slipped, move it to its proper place by using good body mechanics.

9. Ask the client to turn onto his side toward the side rail and move as close to the rail as possible. If he cannot turn, have him stay on his back and move as close to the side rail as possible.
10. Adjust the pillow. Check it for dentures, glasses, money, etc.
11. Fold the cotton draw sheet toward the client, and tuck it in against his back. Protect him from any soiled matter on the bedding.
12. Raise the plastic draw sheet toward the client, and tuck it in against his back.
13. Roll the bottom sheet toward the client, and tuck it against his back. This strips your side of the bed down to the mattress.

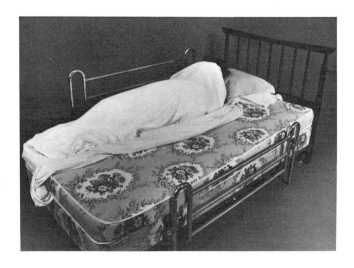

14. Take the large clean sheet and fold it lengthwise. Place it on the bed, still folded, with the fold running along the middle of the mattress. The small hem end of the sheet should be even with the bottom of the mattress. Roll the top half of the sheet toward the client. (This is for the

other side of the bed.) Tuck the folds against his back.
15. Tuck the sheet around the head of the bed by raising the mattress with the hand closest to the foot of the bed and tucking with the other hand.
16. Miter the corner at the head of the bed. Tuck in the clean bottom sheet on your side from the head to the foot of the mattress.

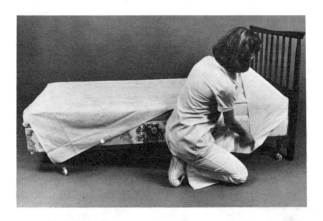

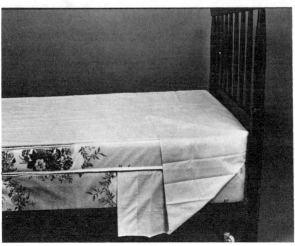

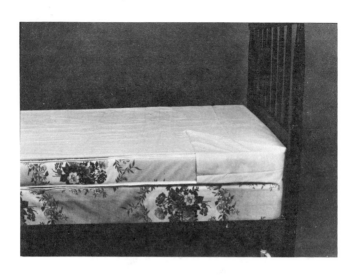

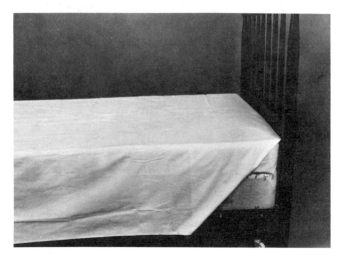

17. Pull the plastic draw sheet toward you, over the clean bottom sheet, and tuck it in.
18. Place the clean draw sheet over the plastic sheet, folded in half. Keep the fold in the center of the bed

near the client. Fold the top half toward the client, tucking the folds under his back, as you did with the bottom sheet. Tuck the free edge of the draw sheet under the mattress.

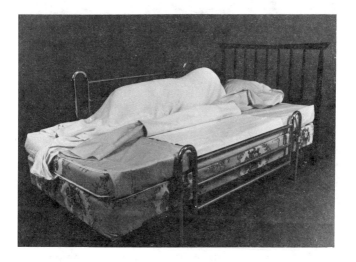

19. Ask or help the client, to roll over the "hump" onto the clean sheets toward you. Raise the side rails on your side and lock them. Go to the opposite side of the bed.
20. Lower the side rails. Remove the old bottom sheet and cotton draw sheet. Put them into the container for soiled linen. Pull the fresh bottom sheet toward the edge of the bed and tuck it in. Be sure it is free of wrinkles.
21. One at a time, pull and tuck each draw sheet under the mattress.
22. Have the client turn on his back.
23. Change the pillowcase and reposition the pillow.
24. Spread the clean top sheet over the bath blanket with the wide hem to the top. Ask the client to hold the hem of the sheet as you remove the bath blanket. If he cannot hold it, tuck the sheet under his shoulders.

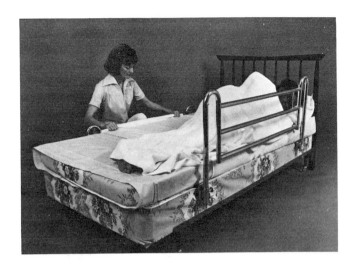

25. Spread the blanket over the top sheet. Tuck the blanket and top sheet in at the foot of the bed by making a mitred corner. Be sure the top covers are loose enough so the client can move his feet. Pull up the side rails.
26. Go to the other side of the bed. Pull down the side rails and miter the top sheet and blanket.
27. Make a cuff by folding the top sheet over the blanket. Reposition the client and leave him in a safe comfortable position.

Safety and Fire Protection

Make yourself aware of the potential hazards in the home and work to remedy them if possible. More accidents occur in the home than in any other place. Be careful! Be aware! Be alert!

- Keep the telephone numbers of the police, rescue squad, fire department, and poison control center near each telephone.

- Do not reach into the trash or garbage. You may hurt yourself on sharp objects.
- Know how to get out of the house in case of fire and how to help your client out in a safe manner.
- Discuss emergency communication with your supervisor. If there is no telephone available, determine what is the best route of communicating.
- Report any unsafe situation to your supervisor.
- Do not attempt a task if you have any doubt that you can do it.

Safety Precautions for Children

- Small children should never be left unattended when they are awake.
- Articles used in the child's care should be kept out of reach of a toddler when they are not being used. Watch especially for needles, water, safety pins, medication, matches, and electrical equipment.
- Toys should be put away and never left on stairs or in places where people may trip on them.
- The sides of a child's crib should be up at all times except when someone is giving direct care to the child.
- Doors to stairways and the kitchen should be closed and locked.
- Venetian blind cords should be kept out of reach of children.
- Be sure there are no small toys or objects in the bed or crib that a child could swallow.
- Be sure there are no large objects in the bed/crib that the child could stand on and fall out.
- Keep all poisonous substances in a high place behind locked doors.

Safety Precautions for the Aged

- Be sure there is adequate lighting for every task.

- Be alert to sensory changes that may have taken place.
- Protect your client from falling.
- Protect your client from burns.
- If a confused client tells you he is going to do something that you know is harmful, take him seriously and protect him.
- Protect your client against extreme hot and cold temperatures.

Electricity

- Make sure all electrical equipment you use is in good condition.
- Be sure all cords are in good condition and that you are using the proper tool for the proper task.

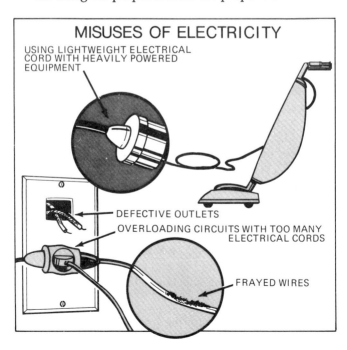

MISUSES OF ELECTRICITY

USING LIGHTWEIGHT ELECTRICAL CORD WITH HEAVILY POWERED EQUIPMENT

DEFECTIVE OUTLETS

OVERLOADING CIRCUITS WITH TOO MANY ELECTRICAL CORDS

FRAYED WIRES

- Do not put electrical cords under rugs. They get frayed and can go unnoticed under the rugs. This is a perfect place for a fire to start.
- Be sure your hands are dry before you touch any piece of electrical equipment.
- Do not change fuses or touch electrical circuit breakers unless you are sure you know what you are doing.
- Do not run all household appliances at the same time in an effort to save time.

Smoking

Many clients smoke. Many visitors smoke. If a client permits smoking in his house unless it is not allowed due to medical reasons or the presence of oxygen, you will be asked to tolerate it. If you are uncomfortable in a house where there is cigarette smoke, discuss this with your supervisor.

- Be sure that ashtrays are provided and used.
- Never empty warm ashtrays into plastic bags, plastic wastebaskets, or plastic containers. Wet the ashes if they feel warm.
- A client who has been given a sedative should not smoke.
- A confused client should not smoke.
- A client in bed should not smoke unattended.
- Check chairs, upholstery, and blankets for ashes or cigarettes if your client is smoking.
- If a client has hand tremors, light his cigarette and assist the client in smoking.

Safety in the Kitchen

- Keep a fire extinguisher in the kitchen.
- Do not leave grease on the stove. Clean it up.

- Do not put water on a grease fire. Use a chemical fire extinguisher or throw baking soda on it to smother the flames.
- Do not leave cooking pots unattended.
- Turn handles of pots away from the edge of the stove.
- Keep paper towels and potholders away from the burners of the stove.
- Store knives so that the blades are protected.
- Electric cooking does not produce a visible flame, so be sure to check that the dial is set at the setting you want or at off.
- If you or your client has a pacemaker, stay out of the kitchen when the microwave oven is working.

Safety in the Bathroom

- Is the toilet secure to the floor? Is the seat secure to the toilet?
- Can your client get up and down safely? Can he sit without support?
- Are the hot and cold faucets correctly marked?
- Is the tub very deep? Can your client get in and out safely?
- Is there ventilation in the bathroom?
- Are the tiles on the floor slippery when wet? Is there a secure bathmat on the floor?
- If there are grab bars, are they secure? Towel bars were not designed to support weight. Do not use them instead of specially designed grab bars.
- If you use electrical equipment such as hair dryers, be sure your feet are dry.

Fire Prevention

Fires start because of

- Smoking and matches
- Improper rubbish disposal

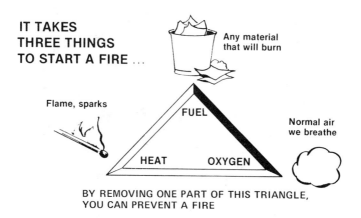

IT TAKES THREE THINGS TO START A FIRE ...

Any material that will burn

Flame, sparks

FUEL

Normal air we breathe

HEAT   OXYGEN

BY REMOVING ONE PART OF THIS TRIANGLE, YOU CAN PREVENT A FIRE

- Misuse of electricity
- Defects in heating systems
- Spontaneous combustion
- Improper cooking techniques
- Improper ventilation

Learn the layout of the house. Ask yourself the following questions:

- Where are the exits from this house in case of fire?
- How would I remove the client from the house?
- Are there fire extinguishers in the house—one for grease fires and one for other types of fires?
- Are there smoke detectors in the house? Do they work?

In case of fire,

- Seal off the fire. If the fire is behind a door, do not open the door. Take another route out of the house. If you must go through a smoke-filled room, wet a cloth and hold it over your mouth and nose. Crawl through the

91

smoke or gas and stay as low to the ground as possible.

- Call the fire department from a neighbor's house. Do not stay in the house for any reason.
- Keep your client warm and comfortable.
- Stay with your client until you know he is safe.

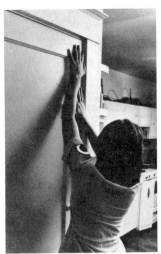

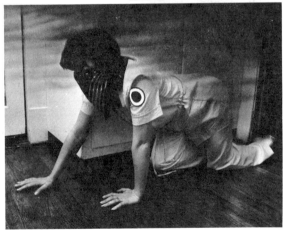

Oxygen Safety

- There is *never* any smoking in a room where an oxygen tank is kept whether or not the tank is in use. Remove cigarettes, matches, and ashtrays from the room.

- Do not use electrical equipment such as hair dryers, electrical heating pads, or shavers near oxygen. Keep the plugs out of the walls while the oxygen is running.
- Do not use candles or open flames in the room.
- Avoid combing the client's hair while he is receiving oxygen. A spark of electricity from his hair can cause a fire.
- Do not use oil, rubbing alcohol, or talcum powder while the client is receiving oxygen. Do not use wool, nylon, or synthetic fabrics in the room. Use cotton whenever possible.
- All oxygen tanks are painted green.
- Do not touch the valves and dials on the oxygen equipment.

Making Your Own Equipment

Backrest

A backrest is used to prop a client up in bed while he eats, takes part in his care, or visits with people. When a client is propped up, it is important that

- He should be able to support himself in that position and not fall to one side or out of bed.
- He should be able to call for help or to change his position.
- The position should be permitted by the physician.
- You should be able to secure the backrest so it does not slip in the bed.

Procedure: Making a Backrest

1. Gather the equipment you will need: a clean sturdy, cardboard box about 24 inches by 24 inches by 18

inches, a pair of scissors or sharp knife, and string, tape, or cord to secure the ends.

2. Position the box on a flat surface with the side toward you.

3. Cut the right and left seams from the top to the bottom. The box will now be open, and the front will be lying flat.

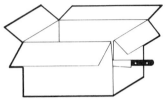

4. Make a cut (score) through the inside layer of the cardboard on the side flaps as shown in the figure.

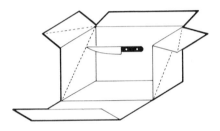

5. Fold the ends toward the middle of the box along the scoring lines.

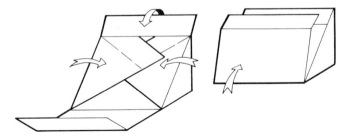

6. Fold up the front of the box (the part that has been lying flat) to cover the triangles.

7. Fold the top down and tie or tape.

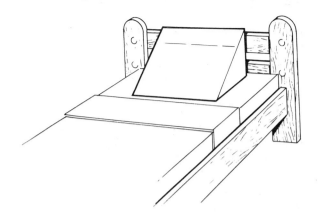

Bed Tables

A bed table can be used by the client during meal time, during personal care, and for recreation activities. A table at the side of the bed, much like the ones in a hospital, can be made by standing an adjustable ironing board near the bed, adjusting the height, and locking it into place.

Procedure: Making a Bed Table

1. Gather the equipment you will need: clean, sturdy cardboard box about 10 inches by 12 inches by 24 inches, a sharp knife or pair of scissors, a pencil.
2. Cut off the four top flaps of the box along the seams.

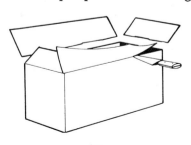

3. Draw a curved opening on both wide sides of the box. Be sure the opening is large enough to fit over the client's legs. Be sure there is enough cardboard left, at least 2 inches, on the side to support the weight of the items that will be put on the bed table.

4. Cut out the opening along the lines you have drawn.

5. Cut small openings in the side near the top for handholds.

6. Cover the table with adhesive-backed plastic or wallpaper to protect it and make it more attractive.

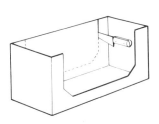

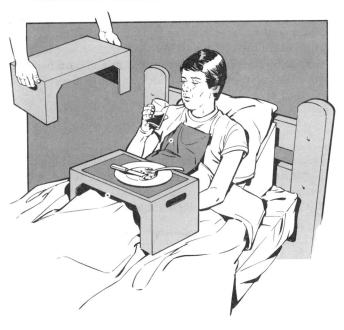

Bed Cradle

This is used under the blankets and sheets and over the client's legs so that the covers do not touch the skin. Use the same procedure to make a bed cradle as you would to make a bed table. Be sure, however, that the box is big enough to provide space for the client's legs to move.

Foot Board

This is used to support the covers so they do not touch the client's toes and to provide a place where the client can rest his feet. If the possibility of foot drop exists, this is a very necessary piece of equipment.

Procedure: Making a Footboard

1. Gather the equipment you will need: a piece of wood about as long as the bed is wide and high enough to keep the covers at least 2 inches off the client's feet, a piece of board about the same size to slip under the mattress, 2 blocks of wood for added support, sandpaper, nails or screws, hammer or screwdriver.
2. Sand the edges of the boards so that they are smooth and will not cause splinters or tear the bedcovers.

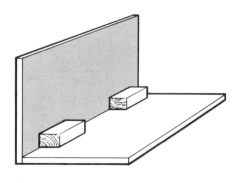

3. Secure the two pieces of wood at right angles to each other.
4. Secure the supports as illustrated.
5. Position the footboard on the bed under the bed covers.
6. Instruct the client and family how to use the footboard.

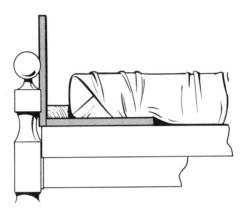

8

Planning, Purchasing, and Serving Food

BASIC NUTRITION

Good nutrition is especially important for a person whose body is in a weakened condition. Food is converted into energy to carry out the day's activities and is used by the body to rebuild body tissue. Eating is also a social activity.

All foods have been divided into *four basic food groups:* milk; vegetables and fruit; meat and fish; and breads, cereals, and potatoes. By eating the correct number of servings from each food group, a person gets the correct amount of each nutrient. A *nutrient* is a substance necessary for the body to repair, maintain, and grow new cells.

PLANNING, SHOPPING, AND SERVING A MEAL

Let the client take an active part in developing his menu and meal schedule. Some people eat three meals a day, and some prefer to snack all day long. Discuss with the client his preference.

NUTRIENT CLASS	BODILY FUNCTION	FOOD SOURCES
CARBOHYDRATES	Provides work energy for body activities, and heat energy for maintenance of body temperature.	Cereal grains and their products (bread, breakfast cereals, macaroni products), potatoes, sugar, syrups, fruits, milk, vegetables, nuts.
PROTEINS	Build and renew body tissues; regulate body functions and supply energy. Complete proteins: maintain life and provide growth. Incomplete proteins: maintain life but do not provide for growth.	Complete proteins: Derived from animal foods—meat, milk, eggs, fish, cheese, poultry. Incomplete proteins: Derived from vegetable foods—soybeans, dry beans, peas, some nuts and whole grain products.
FATS	Give work energy for body activities and heat energy for maintenance of body temperature. Carrier of vitamins A and D, provide fatty acids necessary for growth and maintenance of body tissues.	Some foods are chiefly fat, such as lard, vegetable fats and oils, and butter. Many other foods contain smaller proportions of fats—nuts, meats, fish, poultry, cream, whole milk.

NUTRIENT CLASS	BODILY FUNCTION	FOOD SOURCES
MINERALS **Calcium** 	Builds and renews bones, teeth, and other tissues; regulates the activities of the muscles, heart, nerves; and controls the clotting of blood.	Milk and milk products, except butter; most dark green vegetables; canned salmon.
Phosphorus 	Associated with calcium in some functions needed to build and renew bones and teeth. Influences the oxidation of foods in the body cells; important in nerve tissue.	Widely distributed in foods; especially cheese, oat cereals, whole-wheat products, dry beans and peas, meat, fish, poultry, nuts.
Iron 	Builds and renews hemoglobin, the red pigment in blood which carries oxygen from the lungs to the cells.	Eggs, meat, especially liver and kidney; deep-yellow and dark green vegetables; potatoes, dried fruits, whole-grain products; enriched flour, bread, breakfast cereals.

NUTRIENT CLASS	BODILY FUNCTION	FOOD SOURCES
MINERALS *(cont.)* **Iodine**	Enables the thyroid gland to perform its function of controling the rate at which foods are oxidized in the cells.	Fish (obtained from the sea), some plant foods grown in soils containing iodine; table salt fortified with iodine (iodized).
VITAMINS A	Necessary for normal functioning of the eyes, prevents night blindness. Ensures a healthy condition of the skin, hair, and mucous membranes. Maintains a state of resistance to infection of the eyes, mouth, and respiratory tract.	One form of Vitamin A is yellow and one form is colorless. Apricots, cantaloupe, milk, cheese, eggs, meat organs, (especially liver and kidney), fortified margarine, butter, fish-liver oils, dark green and deep yellow vegetables.
B Complex B₁ (Thiamine)	Maintains a healty condition of the nerves. Fosters a good appetite. Helps the body cells use carbohydrates.	Whole-grain and enriched grain products; meats (especially pork, liver, and kidney). Dry beans and peas.

NUTRIENT CLASS	BODILY FUNCTION	FOOD SOURCES
VITAMINS (*cont.*) B₂ (Riboflavin)	Keeps the skin, mouth, and eyes in a healty condition. Acts with other nutrients to form enzymes and control oxidation in cells.	Milk, cheese, eggs, meat (especially liver and kidney), whole grain and enriched grain products, dark green vegetables.
Niacin	Influences the oxidation of carbohydrates and proteins in the body cells.	Liver, meat, fish, poultry, eggs, peanuts; dark green vegetables, whole-grain and enriched cereal products.
B₁₂	Regulates specific processes in digestion. Helps maintain normal functions of muscles, nerves, heart, blood—general body metabolism.	Liver, other organ meats, cheese, eggs, milk, leafy green vegetables.

NUTRIENT CLASS	BODILY FUNCTION	FOOD SOURCES
VITAMINS (cont.) **C (Ascorbic Acid)** 	Acts as a cement between body cells, and helps them work together to carry out their special functions. Maintains a sound condition of bones, teeth, and gums. Not stored in the body.	Fresh, raw citrus fruits and vegetables—oranges, grapefruit, cantaloupe, strawberries, tomatoes, raw onions, cabbage, green and sweet red peppers, dark green vegetables.
D 	Enables the growing body to use calcium and phosphorus in a normal way to build bones and teeth.	Provided by Vitamin D fortification of certain foods, such as milk and margarine. Also fish-liver oils and eggs. Sunshine is also a source of Vitamin D.
WATER 	Regulates body processes. Aids in regulating body temperature. Carries nutrients to body cells and carries waste products away from them. Helps to lubricate joints. Water has no food value, although most water contains mineral elements. More immediately necessary to life than food—second only to oxygen.	Drinking water, and other beverages; all foods except those made up of a single nutrient, as sugar and some fats. Milk, milk drinks, soups, vegetables, fruit juices, ice cream, watermelon, strawberries, lettuce, tomatoes, cereals, other dry products.

Food habits can be influenced by religious beliefs and ethnic backgrounds. Some clients do not eat pork products or meat. Some do not mix certain foods together. Discuss the dietary practices with the family before you plan the menu and before you shop for food.

As you make out your shopping list, take into consideration the ingredients the client has on hand and the menus you have planned.

- *Variety.* No one food is perfect. A well-balanced diet consists of foods from all four food groups.
- *Texture.* Unless the client is on a special diet, try to choose foods with different textures within the same meal.
- *Flavors.* Prepare a variety of flavors. Keep the strong flavored foods as the spotlight of the meal and the milder flavored foods as the background.
- *Temperature.* Ask the client at what temperature he likes his food served.
- *Taste.* Cook the meal to the taste of the client. Discuss with the family the spices they like in their food.
- *Shape.* Ask the family how they like their food cut: in chunks, sliced, or mashed.
- *Color.* Keep colors compatible. Add accents such as parsley, olives, radishes, or carrot curls.
- *Cost.* Plan meals that are within the client's budget.

Read the labels to determine the amount of salt, sugar, or other restricted items in every container. Labels also provide information about the amount of food in the container, the number of servings in the container, and the number of calories per serving. Products that contain more than one ingredient must list all ingredients used in the making of the product with the product used most listed first.

UNIT PRICING

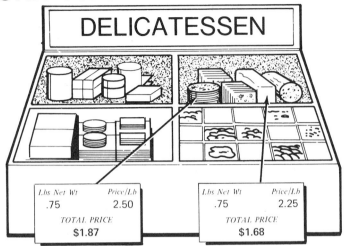

DELICATESSEN

Lbs Net Wt	Price/Lb
.75	2.50
TOTAL PRICE	
$1.87	

Lbs Net Wt	Price/Lb
.75	2.25
TOTAL PRICE	
$1.68	

Comparing prices before you buy helps you save!
Chunk salami is usually cheaper than bulk sliced.
Bulk sliced is usually cheaper than vacuum packed.

Most stores display prices by unit. *Unit pricing* tells the customer what the cost of the item is by a particular quantity: per pound, per quart, or per dozen.

Before you go shopping,

- Prepare a list and discuss it with your client.
- Discuss the size of the purchase, money available, likes and dislikes, and favorite stores. These are the client's choice. Be guided by them. Discuss with your supervisor if you feel the client is not spending his money wisely.
- Discuss the size of items your client prefers. Does he always buy the large size or the medium size? Does he prefer a special brand of an item?

- Be sure your client will be safe while you are out.

After you shop,

- Save all receipts.
- Carefully write down how much money you were given, how much you spent, and how much change you brought back.

When buying foods high in protein, you can reduce the cost by

- Using poultry when it is cheaper than meat
- Considering cuts of meat that may cost more per pound but give more servings per person
- Learning to prepare less tender cuts of meats in casseroles or pot roasts
- Using fillers such as bread crumbs or pasta to make meat dishes serve more people

Storing Food

- Do not buy more food than you can safely store.
- Keep refrigerators operating properly by defrosting when needed.
- Check the expiration date on food before purchasing. Use food with the shortest shelf life first.
- Dry ingredients such as flour, sugar, cereal, and pasta products should be stored in tightly covered containers.
- *Meats.* Refrigerate all meats. Ground meat and variety meats spoil more quickly than others, so use them soon after purchase.
- *Fruits and vegetables.* Keep most fruits and vegetables in the refrigerator in plastic bags, tightly covered containers, or the crisper.
- *Bread.* If wrapped properly, bread can be frozen to keep it most efficiently for a long time.

- *Milk.* Instant nonfat dry milk can be used in many of the same ways as whole milk and can be stored for much longer periods of time without refrigeration.
- *Canned foods.* Store cans in a cool, dry place. Do not use any can that has a top or bottom than can be pushed in. This could mean the can is no longer sealed and its contents are spoiled.
- *Frozen foods.* Keep in freezer at 0 °F temperature until ready to use.

Methods of Cooking

- *Bake or roast:* to cook with dry heat in a confined space, such as an oven.
- *Boil:* to cook in a liquid that is hot enough for bubbles to break the surface.
- *Braise:* a long, slow-cooking method that makes use of moist heat in a tightly covered vessel at a temperature just below boiling. The cooking liquid should just barely cover the food to be braised. Braising is a good way to cook tough meats and vegetables, as the long cooking breaks down the fibers.
- *Broil:* to cook directly under or over a source of heat.
- *Fry:* to cook food in fat or oil. When only a small amount of fat is used, the process is called pan frying or sautéing. When enough fat is used to cover the food, the process is called deep frying or deep-fat frying.
- *Poach:* a method of cooking used to preserve the delicate texture and prevent the toughening of food. The food is covered by water or some other liquid. Depending on the type of food being cooked, the liquid may be either at a boil or slightly below the boiling point.
- *Steam:* a method of cooking in which the food is exposed to the steam of boiling water. The food must be above the liquid, never in it. The container is kept closed during cooking to let the steam accumulate.

Steaming keeps a high proportion of the original flavor and texture of the foods because the nutrients are not dissolved in the cooking liquid.

- *Stew:* a process of long, slow cooking of food in liquid in a covered pot with seasoning. This process is good for tougher cuts of meat.

Serving a Meal

- Tell the client you will be serving him a meal.
- Offer the client the bedpan or urinal before he eats.
- Offer the client oral hygiene before and after the meal.
- Most people enjoy company during a meal. Visitors and family members should be encouraged to remain with the client.
- Ask the client where he would prefer eating.
- Discuss with the client the order in which he prefers his food. Some people prefer their salads before their main course; others eat it after.

Mealtime observations

- Does the client have a good appetite?
- Does the client eat food on his diet?
- Does the client have any discomfort associated with eating?
- Does the client drink enough fluids?
- Who serves the client when you are not in the house?

THERAPEUTIC DIETS

A *therapeutic diet* is one which is prescribed by the physician to meet specific medical needs of the client. This diet will be planned to incorporate the client's likes and dislikes, his ethnic background, and his budget. If you notice that a client is not maintaining his diet, or if he has questions, call your supervisor.

Types of Diets Given to Patients: What They Are and Why They Are Used

Type of Diet	Description	Common Purpose	Foods often Recommended	Foods to Avoid
Normal Regular	Provides all essentials of good nourishment in normal forms	For clients who do not need special diets		
Soft (mechanical)	Same foods as on a normal diet, but chopped or strained	For clients who have difficulty in chewing or swallowing		
Bland	Foods mild in flavor and easy to digest; omits spicy foods	Avoids irritation of the digestive tract, as with ulcer and colitis clients	Puddings, creamed dishes, milk, eggs, plain potatoes	Fried foods, raw vegetables or fruit, whole-grain products
Low residue	Foods low in bulk; omits foods difficult to digest	Spares the lower digestive tract, as with clients having rectal disease		Whole-grain products, uncooked fruits and vegetables
High calorie	Foods high in protein, minerals, and vitamins	For underweight or malnourished clients	Eggnog, ice cream, frequent snacks, peanut butter, milk	

Type of Diet	Description	Common Purpose	Foods often Recommended	Foods to Avoid
Low calorie	Low in cream, butter, cereals, deserts, and fats	For clients who should lose weight	Skim milk, fresh fruit and vegetables, lean meat, fish	Fried foods, sauces, gravies, rich desserts
Diabetic	Balance of carbohydrates, protein, and fats, devised according to the needs of individual clients	For diabetic clients: matches food intake with the insulin and nutritional requirements	Fresh fruits and vegetables, low-sugar products	High-sugar foods, alcohol, carbonated beverages
High protein	Meal supplemented with high-protein foods, such as meat, fish, cheese, milk, and eggs	Assists in the growth and repair of tissues wasted by disease	Milk, meat, eggs, cheese, fish	
Low fat	Limited amounts of butter, cream, fats, and eggs	For clients who have difficulty digesting fats as in gall-bladder, cardiovascular, and liver disturbances	Veal, poultry, fish, skim milk, fresh fruits and vegetables	Bacon, butter, cheese, fried foods, liver, whole milk, ice cream, chocolate
Low cholesterol	Low in eggs, whole milk, and meats	Helps regulate the amount of cholesterol in the blood	Fruits, vegetables, cereals, grains, nuts, vegetable oil	Brains, organ meats

CHEMOTHERAPY AND RADIATION

Many people who are receiving chemotherapy and radiation therapy change their eating habits due to nausea, appetite loss, and/or constipation. Some helpful hints during these times are

- Decrease intake of red meat and increase intake of fish, chicken, and other foods high in protein.
- Use plastic utensils, as some people complain of a bitter taste from metal utensils.
- Maintain adequate fluid intake of cool liquids.
- Eat small, frequent meals; chew food well; eat warm, not hot food.
- Decrease intake of sweets and fried foods.
- Remain in a sitting position for at least two hours after meals.
- Eat non-gas producing foods.
- Discuss the fiber intake with your supervisor.
- Provide a pleasant, quiet atmosphere during mealtimes.
- Vary the diet.

FEEDING A CLIENT

It may be difficult for an adult to accept the idea of not being able to feed himself. Encourage him to do as much as he can, and only give assistance when needed. Talk pleasantly to him, but not too much. Be friendly and natural. Be sure the client can swallow both solid and liquid foods before you put the food into his mouth. Pay special attention to the temperature of foods and liquids. If a client is blind, name each mouthful before you offer it to him.

- Do not rush the feeding. Sit if possible.
- Be gentle with forks and spoons; straws may help during the feeding of liquids.
- Feed the foods separately rather than mixed together.
- When offering a glass or cup, first touch it to the client's lips.
- Note the client's intake and output. Record if necessary.
- Note your observations about the client. Record if necessary.

9

Basic Body Movement and Positions

BODY MECHANICS

Body mechanics refers to the way of standing and moving one's body so as to prevent injury, avoid fatigue, and make the best use of strength. Proper body mechanics is a major safety factor both for you and your client. The muscles that flex the joints are generally the strongest ones. Your strongest muscles are in your arms and your legs, not your back. By slightly bending your arms and your back when doing a heavy job, you are putting your muscles in the best position to accomplish the work.

Your *base of support* determines how stable you are. The larger the base of support, the more stable you are, the better you are able to work, and the safer you are.

The *center of gravity* of any object is the point at which, when held, you will have the greatest control over the object with the least amount of effort. A person's center of gravity is in the pelvic area. When holding or assisting a client, you will have the greatest control, and the client will feel safest, if you hold him close to his center of gravity.

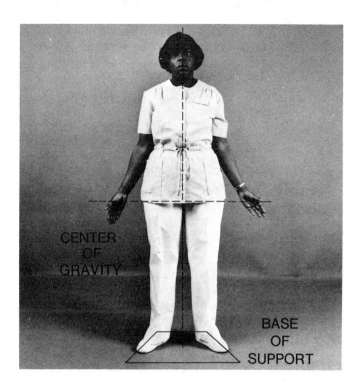

CENTER
OF
GRAVITY

BASE
OF
SUPPORT

Balancing is the process of keeping your center of gravity within your base of support. This is necessary when you are lifting a heavy object, when you make a bed, and when a client gets up from a sitting position. By spreading your feet and bending your knees, you lower your center of gravity and keep it within your base of support. When a client gets up from a sitting position, he must bend forward enough so that his center of gravity is balanced over his base of support.

- As you are working, use as many muscle groups as possible.
- Use both hands rather than only one hand.

115

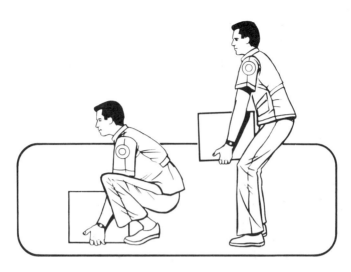

- Use good posture. Keep your body aligned properly. Keep your back straight. Have your knees bent. Keep your weight evenly balanced over both feet.
- When lifting an object your feet should be at least 12 inches apart to give you the best base of support. You should be as close to the load that is being lifted as possible.
- When moving a heavy object, push it rather than pull it, roll it rather than carry it.
- If you think you may not be able to accomplish a task safely, do not start it. Get help.
- Lift smoothly. Always count, "one, two, three" with the other person with whom you are working. Do this with both the client and with other helpers.
- When you want to change the direction of movement,
  —pivot with your feet,
  —turn with short steps,
  —turn with your whole body without twisting your neck and back.

- Use your arms to support an object; the muscles of your legs actually do the lifting, not the muscles in your back.
- When you are doing work such as making a bed or exercising a client, work with the direction of your effort.
- When working with a client who is not in a hospital bed, put one foot on the lowest side rail or on a foot stool to relieve the pressure on your back.

CLIENT'S DAILY LEVEL OF ABILITY

Check your *client's daily level of ability* each day before you start an activity. An activity performed one day may not be possible the next day.

- Can the client hear and understand you?
- Can the client follow directions?
- How much can the client do alone?
- What are the client's vital signs?
- Will pain be a factor in this activity?
- Are joint motions limited?
- Does the client tire easily?

Assisting Clients

- Know your own capabilities.
- Expect the client to do as much as possible. Help only when needed.
- Work at the client's level and speed.
- Direct activity instead of asking for it. For example, tell the client, "It is time to stand, Mrs. C.," instead of, "Do you want to stand up?"
  If the client says no, what will you do?
- Give short, clear directions.

- Plan ahead. Gather all equipment before you begin an activity.
- Praise the client for following directions. If he does not do it correctly, stop the activity and redirect him until the correct activity is done. This way, the client will get used to doing the activity the correct way and will not develop any bad habits.
- Your body language will be noticed by the client. Make sure your nonverbal messages fit the words you use.
- Touch is the most important sense. You will be giving a great deal of physical contact to your client. If you are comfortable touching him, he will be comfortable too.
- Avoid sudden, jerky movements. Use smooth, steady motions.

POSITIONING A CLIENT IN BED

The correct positioning of a body is referred to as *body alignment*. Proper alignment is necessary when standing, when sitting, and when lying in bed. It is often necessary to use pillows and towels to keep the alignment of a client correct when they are lying in bed. If a client is able to maintain his own alignment, he should be encouraged to do so. If he is unable to do this, however, it is your responsibility to see that the proper position is maintained.

Clients who have a weakness or type of disability often need physical therapy and assistance with some movements. The side of their body that is weakened, should not be called "the bad side"; refer to it as the *involved side*. Point out to your client the positive aspects of his care and encourage him. The term *functional* describes the usefulness of something and usually produces a desired result. It may be an activity or a body part. An activity such as brushing one's hair is a functional activity. *Nonfunctional* body parts will not perform a useful activity.

Moving a Client in Bed

To move a client who cannot move easily in bed, use a *pull sheet*. A pull sheet can be the draw sheet, the bottom sheet, or an extra sheet folded over several times and placed under the client for this specific purpose. This is usually done by two people. Roll up the sheet tightly next to the client's body. Grip the edges underhand to slide the client into the desired position. By using the sheet, you avoid friction and irritation to the client's skin.

The position of your client will depend on the following:

- The client's preference
- The client's diagnosis
- Doctor's orders
- Safety

Positioning a Client Who Has a Weak Side on His Back

- Place a small pillow under the client's head.
- Place a small hand towel under the shoulder blade of the weak side, fold a bath towel under the hip of the weak side, roll a washcloth up in the hand of the weak side.
- Support the arm and elbow on a pillow above the heart.
- Place a small pillow under the calf of the weak leg.
- Allow the heels to hang off the mattress.
- Loosen the top sheet so pressure is removed from the toes.

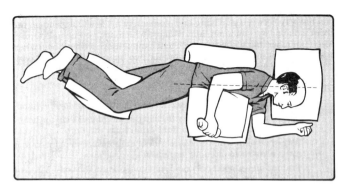

Positioning a Client on His Uninvolved Side

- Place a small pillow under the head, keeping the head in alignment with the spine.
- Roll a large pillow lengthwise and tuck it in at the client's back for support and to prevent him from rolling.
- Place a pillow in front and under the arm to keep it the same height as the shoulder. Place a medium pillow between the client's knees with the top knee slightly bent or with both knees bent. Place a small pillow between the two ankles and the feet to prevent two skin surfaces from rubbing together.
- Change the client's position at least every two hours. Check the client frequently to be sure he is comfortable.

Positioning a Client on His Involved Side

- Use the same principles as above.
- Change the client's position more frequently. With disability can come a lessened sense of pain and pressure.

Procedure: Moving the Client up in Bed with His Help

1. Tell the client you are going to help him move up in bed.

2. Lock the wheels of the bed. Raise the bed to the height best for you.
3. Lower the side rail on your side. Leave the side rail up on the other side. Remove the pillow.
4. Put one hand under the client's shoulder and the other under his buttocks.
5. Tell the client to bend his knees with feet firmly braced against the mattress. The client's hands should be on the mattress also.
6. Stand with your feet 12 inches apart. The foot closest to the head of the bed should be pointed in that direction. Bend your knees. Keep your back straight. Bend your body from the hips, facing the client and turning slightly toward the head of the bed.

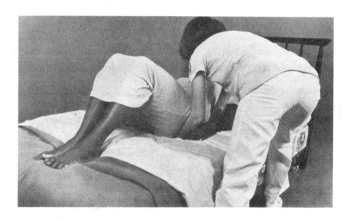

7. At the signal "one, two, three," have the client pull with his hand toward the head of the bed, and pushing with his feet against the mattress.
8. At the same time, help the client move toward the head of the bed by sliding him with your hands and arms. Reposition the pillow. Make sure the client is comfortable. Raise the side rails.

Procedure: Moving a Client Up in Bed
(Two People)

1. Tell the client you and your partner are going to move
   him up in the bed. Say this even if the client appears
   to be unconscious.
2. Lock the wheels of the bed. Raise the bed to the height
   best for you.
3. Remove the pillow. Position yourself on one side of
   the bed and your helper on the other. Lower the side
   rails on both sides.
4. Both of you should stand slightly turned toward the
   head of the bed with your feet 23 inches apart. The foot
   closest to the head of the bed should be pointed in that
   direction. Bend your knees. Keep your backs straight.
5. Use of a draw sheet or pull sheet is always preferred.
   Roll the draw sheet up to the client's body and grab
   underhand. You and your partner should shift your
   weight from your back legs to the legs pointed toward

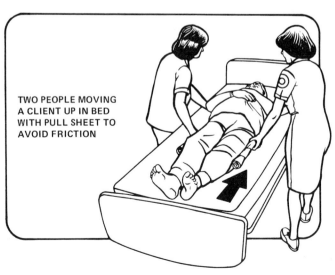

TWO PEOPLE MOVING
A CLIENT UP IN BED
WITH PULL SHEET TO
AVOID FRICTION

the head of the bed. As you do this, lock your arms and backs in position. The client will move as you do. At the signal "one, two, three," both you and your partner move the client by shifting your weight.

6. Put the pillow back in place. Make sure the client is comfortable. Raise the side rails.

Procedure: Moving a Client Up in Bed (One Person)

1. Tell the client you are going to move him up in the bed. Say this even if the client appears to be unconscious.

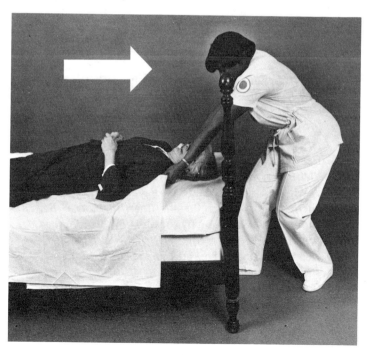

2. Lock the wheels of the bed. Raise the bed to the height best for you.
3. Remove the pillow. Stand at the head of the bed. One foot should be close to the bed, the other slightly behind.
4. Reach over the top of the draw sheet. Roll the edge and grab it.
5. On the count of "one, two, three" lock your arms and back and shift your weight to your back leg. The client will slide easily to the top of the bed on the sheet.
6. Put the pillow back in place. Make sure the client is comfortable. Raise the side rails.

Procedure: Moving a Client to One Side of the Bed on His Back

1. Tell the client you are going to move him up in the bed. Say this even if the client appears to be unconscious.
2. Lock the wheels of the bed. Raise the bed to the height best for you.
3. Remove the pillow. Lower the side rail on your side.
4. Place your feet so that one is close to the bed, the other is slightly behind. Slide both your arms under the client's back to his far shoulder. Slide the client's shoulders toward you by rocking your weight to your back foot.
5. Keep your knees bent and your back straight as you slide the client.
6. Repeat this procedure under the client's buttocks.
7. Put the pillow back in place. Make sure the client is comfortable. Raise the side rails.

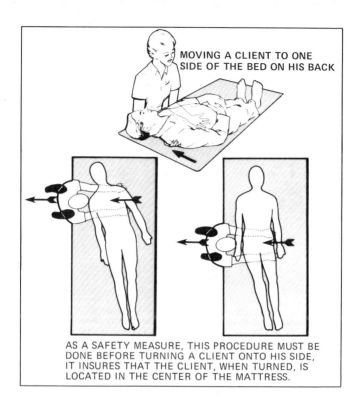

MOVING A CLIENT TO ONE
SIDE OF THE BED ON HIS BACK

AS A SAFETY MEASURE, THIS PROCEDURE MUST BE
DONE BEFORE TURNING A CLIENT ONTO HIS SIDE,
IT INSURES THAT THE CLIENT, WHEN TURNED, IS
LOCATED IN THE CENTER OF THE MATTRESS.

Procedure: Rolling a Client Like a Log (Log Rolling)

1. Tell the client you are going to move him up in the bed. Say this even if the client appears to be unconscious.
2. Lock the wheels of the bed. Raise the bed to the height best for you.
3. Remove the pillow. Lower the side rail on your side.
4. Move the client to your side of the bed as in the previous procedure.

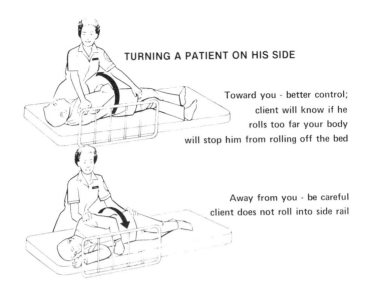

TURNING A PATIENT ON HIS SIDE

Toward you - better control; client will know if he rolls too far your body will stop him from rolling off the bed

Away from you - be careful client does not roll into side rail

5. Raise the side rail on your side of the bed. Go to the other side of the bed and lower the rail.
6. By holding the client at his hip and shoulder, roll the client toward you on to his side.
7. Put the pillow back in place. Make sure the client is comfortable. Raise the side rails.

Procedure: Raising the Client's Head and Shoulders

1. Tell the client you are going to raise his head and shoulders.
2. Lock the wheels of the bed. Raise the bed to the height best for you.
3. Lower the side rail on your side.
4. Slide your arm under the client's shoulder blade. Position your feet 12 inches apart, with one foot pointed

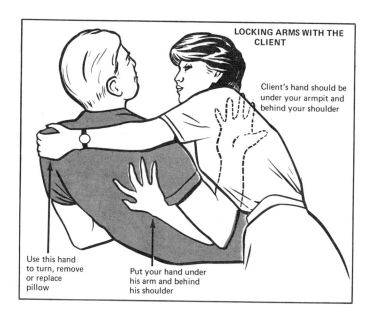

LOCKING ARMS WITH THE CLIENT

Client's hand should be under your armpit and behind your shoulder

Use this hand to turn, remove or replace pillow

Put your hand under his arm and behind his shoulder

toward the foot of the bed. The other foot should be slightly behind. Lock your hands and back and shift your weight from one foot to the other.

5. If the client has some strength, plant your feet in the proper position and let him pull up on you. Hold your arm stationary while the client does the work.

6. Put the pillow back in place. Make sure the client is comfortable. Raise the side rails.

10

Skin Care

BASIC SKIN CARE

Good skin care is one of your prime responsibilities. Inspect the skin daily for changes, reddened areas, tender places, sore areas, or areas of breakdown. By taking corrective action when you notice any changes in the skin, further damage and pain may be prevented. Sometimes the skin will not respond well to your care due to factors beyond your control.

Factors Affecting Skin

- Disease process
- Exercise and mobility
- Medication
- Health habits
- Nutrition
- Financial resources
- Type of care received when you are not in the home

High-Risk Factors

Bony prominences are areas where bones are close to the skin. Pressure on these areas decrease circulation leading to decubitus ulcer formation.

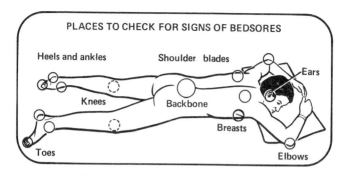

PLACES TO CHECK FOR SIGNS OF BEDSORES

Heels and ankles   Shoulder blades   Ears
Knees   Backbone
Toes   Breasts
Elbows

Obese clients tend to develop decubiti in areas where skin folds rub together causing friction. Check areas under the breasts and between the thighs and the buttocks.

Shearing occurs when the skin is moved one way and the bone and tissue under the skin move another. When this happens, the tiny blood vessels are pinched, and the blood supply to the skin is decreased.

Skin Care of the Elderly

Several changes occur as a person ages:

- Loss of skin tone
- Loss of oils leading to dry, itchy, rough skin
- Loss of underlying layer of fat leading to thin, fragile skin
- Decrease in circulation and the healing process

Ways of Decreasing Pressure to Body Areas

- Use an air cushion. Do not fill it more than half full.
- Place a sheepskin against the skin. Wash it frequently.
- Place an eggcrate mattress under a sheet.
- Position an air mattress or waterfilled mattress between the regular mattress and a sheet. Do not use safety pins.

- Keep sheepskin booties on the client's heels and elbows.

Basic Skin Care

- Be gentle. Do not accidentally scratch the skin.
- Protect the client from the sun, wind, cold, heat, and rain.
- Keep the client clean and dry. Bathing every day is not always necessary, but washing the perineal area with a mild soap daily will prevent odor, skin irritation, and infection. Rinse the skin well.
- Place cornstarch directly on sheets to reduce friction.
- Keep an *incontinent* client clean and dry. Do not use rubber pants. Protect the bed with disposable protectors. Use a plastic draw sheet under a regular sheet.
- Change the client's position at least every two hours.
- Keep linen free of crumbs, hard objects, and wrinkles.
- Be sure clients do not lie on their catheters.

DECUBITUS ULCERS

Signs of a Decubitus Ulcer

A *decubitus ulcer* is an area where the skin has broken because of pressure. Signs of a decubitus area are

- Warm, red, tender, burning areas
- Gray color indicating decreased blood supply
- A blister
- An open wound

Care of a Decubitus Ulcer

Specific treatment must be prescribed by a physician, but you should take the following steps while waiting for more detailed instructions.

Stages of Decubiti Formation

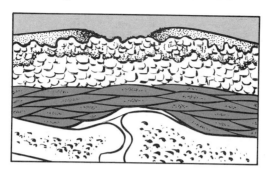

Inflammation or redness of the skin which does not return to normal after 15 minutes of removal of pressure. Edema is present. It involves the epidermis. Skin may or may not be broken.

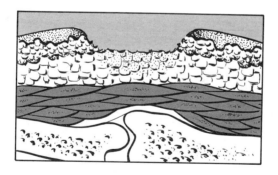

Skin blister or shallow skin ulcer. Involves the epidermis and dermis. Looks like a shallow crater. Area is red, warm, and may or may not have drainage.

Stages of Decubiti Formation (*cont.*)

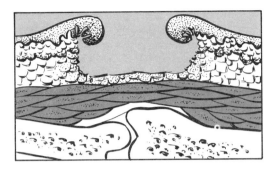

Full thickness skin loss exposing subcutaneous tissue, may extend into next layer. Edema, inflammation, and necrosis present. Drainage present which may or may not have an odor.

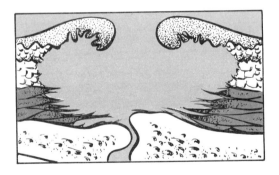

Full-thickness ulcer. Muscle and/or bone can be seen. Infection and necrosis are present. Drainage present, which may or may not have an odor.

- Position the client so that pressure is removed from the area.
- Keep the area clean and dry. This may include the application of a nonsterile dressing.
- Teach the family how to follow the plan of care when you are not there.

BASIC FOOT CARE

Diseases such as COPD, arthritis, diabetes, and hypertension often cause problems due to poor nutrition, lack of circulation, and decreased physical abilities. Be watchful for the following conditions:

- Pain either while resting or during exercise
- Changes in sensation on the skin such as "tingling," "pins and needles," or lack of sensation
- Decreased temperature sensation
- Increased sensitivity to cold
- Increased fluid retention resulting in edema or swelling
- Dry, cracked skin
- Open areas such as blisters or ulcers
- Toenails that are thick and curling under the toes
- Absence of toenails

Basic Foot Care

- Inspect the feet daily for changes.
- Wash and dry feet daily. Use mild soap between the toes. Lubricate dry skin as permitted.
- Do not cut toe nails, bunions, or corns.
- Encourage your client to always wear the proper shoes and stockings that allow the feet to "breathe."
- Do not use garters or rubber bands to hold up socks.
- Protect feet from heat and sand.

RADIATION AND CHEMOTHERAPY: EFFECTS ON THE SKIN

Radiation therapy is the use of a specialized type of energy ray to stop the growth of cancer cells by destroying the cells' ability to grow and reproduce. The lines drawn on the skin by the therapist indicate the target. The side effects of the radiation are the result of the cancer cells and the normal cells being affected.

- Do not wash off the target lines.
- Do not wash the area with soap but with cool water. Keep it free of lotions.
- Protect the area from sunlight with loose-fitting clothes.
- If the area is red, report this. Do not put anything on it.
- Do not use hair removal chemicals or lotions to remove hair as it grows back.

Chemotherapy is a general term used to describe the use of drugs to treat cancer. The drugs destroy the cells' ability to reproduce. The side effects of chemotherapy are the result of the cancer cells and the normal cells being affected.

- If the client's mouth is dry, offer soft, cold bland foods and drink. These will not irritate the mouth.
- Use a soft-bristled toothbrush and nonirritating mouthwash.
- If the hair falls out, use a wig or a hat to protect the scalp. Keep the scalp clean and free of irritation.

11

Personal Care

ORAL HYGIENE

Oral hygiene includes the cleansing of the mouth, gums, and teeth or dentures. This should be done at least twice a day or whenever necessary to decrease a bad taste in the client's mouth, to remove the coating on the tongue, or to decrease odor and help the client feel more refreshed.

Procedure: Oral Hygiene

Be sure the client is able to spit out water before you allow him to put any in his mouth. If the client is able to go to the sink, omit unnecessary steps.

1. Assemble the equipment: fresh water, cup, straw if necessary, toothbrush and tooth paste, emesis basin, small basin or sink, face towel, mouthwash.
2. Have the client sit up. Spread a towel across his chest.
3. Offer the client water to rinse his mouth. Hold the emesis basin under his chin so he can spit out the water.

4. Put toothpaste on the wet toothbrush. Offer the client the toothbrush. Assist him to brush as necessary. Use a gentle motion starting above the gum line and going down the teeth.
5. Offer the client cool water to rinse his mouth. Offer mouthwash.
6. Be sure the client is safe and comfortable. Clean and put away the equipment. Wash your hands.

Dentures

Clients who wear *dentures* require oral hygiene to remove particles of food from the gums and tongue and to stimulate the gums ensuring good circulation. Dentures should be cleaned every 12 hours and soaked in a marked denture cup with cleansing solution when not in the client's mouth. Dentures are expensive and difficult to replace. Do not wrap them in tissue or put them under a pillow where they may be thrown out accidentally.

Procedure: Oral Hygiene for Clients Who Wear Dentures

1. Assemble the equipment: tissues, denture cup, small basin or emesis basin, denture soaking solution, towel, denture toothpaste, mouthwash, soft toothbrush.
2. Spread the towel across the client's chest. Ask him to remove his dentures and place them in the emesis basin lined with a tissue. If the client cannot remove the dentures, assist him.
3. Hold the dentures securely over the sink lined with a towel, washcloth, or paper towel. Fill the sink with water to cushion the dentures if they should slip out of your hands.

4. Apply toothpaste or denture cleanser to the dentures. Brush the dentures until they are clean. *Do not use kitchen cleaner or abrasive cleansers.*
5. Rinse the dentures thoroughly with cool water.
6. Fill the denture cup with denture soaking solution, cool water, or mouthwash. Place the dentures in the cup and cover them.
7. Help the client rinse his mouth and brush his gums with a soft toothbrush.
8. Offer the client his dentures. Be sure they are moist when they are inserted. Leave the labeled denture cup with clean solution easily accessible to the client.
9. Make sure the client is comfortable. Clean and put away the equipment. Wash your hands.

The Unconscious Client

Mouth care for the unconscious client prevents the oral tissues from cracking and bleeding.

Procedure: Oral Hygiene
for the Unconscious Client

Do not put water in the client's mouth. Speak to the client even though it may appear he does not hear you. Do not put your fingers into the client's mouth.

1. Assemble the equipment: towel, small basin or emesis basin, tongue depressor padded with several layers of gauze, lubricant such as glycerine or a solution of glycerine and lemon juice.
2. Turn the client's head toward you supported by a covered pillow.
3. Put a small basin under the client's chin. Wipe the entire mouth and tongue with the padded tongue

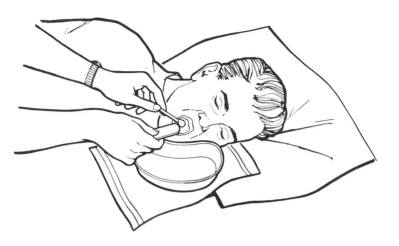

depressor dipped in the glycerine solution. This will leave a protective coating on the oral tissues. Put the used swabs into the basin.

4. Dry the client's face. Put a small amount of lubricant on the lips.
5. Make sure the client is safe and comfortable. Clean and put away the equipment. Wash your hands.

ASSISTING A CLIENT TO DRESS AND UNDRESS

- Allow a client to choose his own clothes. Encourage him to get dressed whenever possible.
- If a client has a safe method of dressing himself do not make any changes.
- Do not expose the client unnecessarily.
- An injured or inflexible arm or leg is first into the garment and last out. To put a shirt on, place the injured arm in the sleeve, put the neck over the client's

head, or bring the shirt around his back. Finally put the arm in the remaining sleeve.
- Inspect the client's feet for blisters or irritated areas when you put on his shoes.

BATHING A CLIENT

- Bathing takes waste products off the skin.
- Bathing cools and refreshes the client.
- Bathing stimulates the skin and improves circulation.
- Bathing requires movement of the muscles.
- Bathing provides a good opportunity for observations.
- Bathing is a social activity.

A client may not need to have a complete bath every day. A partial bath may be all that is necessary. This may be easier for the client, may conserve energy and may offer the most comfort. Some people prefer to bathe in the morning, some in the evening. Discuss with the client his preference and the preference of the physician and family.

Most people are used to bathing themselves and may find your assistance embarrassing. Do not overexpose a client. Protect his modesty.

- Take everything to the bedside before you start a bath.
- When using soap keep it in a soap dish, not the bath water.
- Use lotions and creams the client prefers and that are allowed by the physician.
- Talk to the client as you bathe him.
- Change the bath water as often as necessary so that it remains warm and clean.

- Assist the client with establishing a bathing routine to save his energy.
- Allow the client to bathe as much of his own body as he can safely reach.
- Assist the client in setting up the bathroom or bedroom safely. Then give him privacy.

Procedure: The Complete Bath

1. Assemble the equipment: soap in a soap dish, washcloth, several bath towels, wash basin, powder, deodorant, clean pajamas or gown, bath blanket, orange stick for nail care, lotion for back rub, comb and hairbrush.
2. Position the bed to the highest position. Offer the client a bedpan or urinal.
3. Assist the client with oral hygiene.
4. Remove the blanket and bedspread, leaving the top sheet covering the client. If you are using a bath blanket, replace the top sheet with the bath blanket. Neatly fold the top sheet to be used later.
5. Position the client as flat as is comfortable and close to the side of the bed where you will work. Remove the client's jewelry and nightclothes, keeping the client warm and covered.
6. Fill the wash basin 2/3 full with water at the temperature the client prefers.
7. Put a towel across the client's chest. Using a washcloth wrapped around your hand, wash the client's eyes from the nose to the outside of the face. Wash the rest of the face. Pat the face dry.
8. Place a towel lengthwise under the client's arm farthest from you. Support the arm with the palm of your hand under the elbow. Wash his shoulder, axilla, and arm using long, firm strokes. Rinse the area and pat dry. Place the basin of water on the towel. Support the

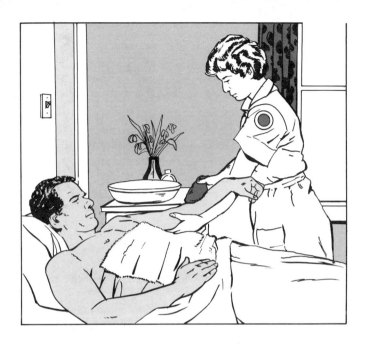

client's hand as you soak it in the basin. Wash the hand and finger nails. Pat them dry and place the entire arm under the bath blanket.

9. Wash the arm and hand closest to you in the same way.
10. Place a towel across the client's chest. Fold the bath blanket down to the client's abdomen. Wash the client's ears, neck, and chest. Be sure and wash under the female client's breasts. Pat the entire area dry. Cover the entire chest with the towel.
11. Fold the bath blanket down to the pubic area. Wash the client's abdomen and navel. Dry the area. Pull the bath blanket up over the chest and remove the towel.
12. Fold the bath blanket back to expose the leg farthest from you. Put a towel lengthwise under the leg. Bending the knee and supporting the leg, wash the leg. If the client can bend his knee easily, put the wash basin

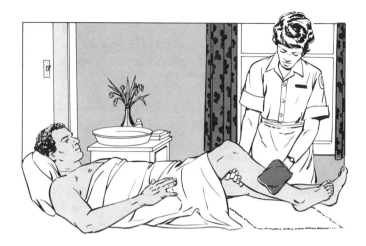

on the towel and soak his feet. Dry the entire leg and foot. Cover them.

13. Wash the leg closest to you in the same manner.
14. Ask the client to turn on his side with his back toward you. Put a towel lengthwise under the client's back. Wash, rinse, and dry his back and buttock area. Give the client a back rub with warm lotion.
15. Have the client turn onto his back. Offer him a soapy washcloth to wash his genital area. Give him a clean, wet washcloth to rinse the genital area. If the client is unable to wash this area, it is your responsibility to do so. Provide for privacy at all times.
16. Dress the client in a clean gown or pajamas. Change the bed if that is appropriate. Make sure the client is safe and comfortable. Clean and put away the equipment. Wash your hands.

Tub Baths

Many clients prefer tub baths to showers. In some cases assisting the client into and out of the tub may be dangerous. Be sure you can perform this safely and that the client's physical condition permits a tub bath.

- Check grab bars in the tub. Do not use towel bars for this purpose.
- Check ventilation in the bathroom. Clients may feel faint from the heat.
- Run the cold water through the faucet last so that if the client touches the faucet, it won't be hot.
- Help the client into the tub. Be sure a nonskid mat is in the tub. Remain close enough so that you can help the client if he calls you.
- Empty the tub before you help the client out of it. Getting out of an empty tub is easier than getting out of a filled one.

Showers

- Be sure the client's physical condition allows him to have a shower. A shower chair placed in the shower may provide needed support.
- Check grab bars in the shower. Do not use soap dishes or towel racks for this purpose.
- Check ventilation in the bathroom. Clients may feel faint from the heat.
- Be sure a nonskid mat is in the shower. Remain close enough so that you can help the client if you are needed.

GIVING A BACK RUB

Rubbing a client's back refreshes and relaxes muscles and stimulates circulation. Back rubs are usually given as part of morning care or any time the client changes position.

A client may not enjoy having his back rubbed. Respect his wishes and do not perform this procedure.

Procedure: Giving a Back Rub

1. Assemble the equipment: towels, lotion of the client's choice, a basin of water.
2. Raise the bed to the highest horizontal position. Ask the client to turn on his side or abdomen. Position him closest to the side of the bed where you are working.
3. Warm the lotion by placing it in the warm basin of water. Warm your hands under warm water.
4. Expose the client's back and buttocks. Apply the lotion to the entire back with the palm of your hands using long, firm strokes from the buttocks to the shoulders and back of the neck and shoulders.
5. Exert firm pressure as you stroke upward from the buttocks toward the shoulders. Use gentle pressure as you move your hands down the back. Do not lift your hands as you massage. Use circular motion on each body area. This rhythmic rubbing motion should continue about three minutes.
6. Dress the client in a clean gown or pajamas. Change the bed if that is appropriate. Make sure the client is safe and comfortable. Clean the equipment. Wash your hands.

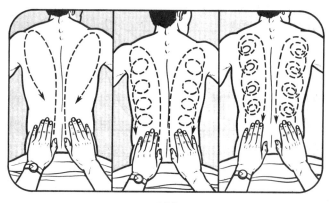

HAIR CARE

Keeping hair neat and clean prevents scalp and hair breakdown, contributes to a sense of wellbeing, improves the circulation in the scalp, and improves appearance.

Before you wash your client's hair, be sure the physician has given permission for this procedure. As you are washing your client's hair, remember to

- Keep the client free of drafts
- Never cut or color the client's hair
- Never give the client a permanent
- Never use a hot comb or curling iron on the client's hair
- Style the client's hair as he or she usually wears it

Procedure: Giving the Client a Shampoo in Bed

1. Assemble the equipment: comb and brush, shampoo, conditioner (optional), several containers of warm to hot water, chair, pitcher, large basin or pail, bed protectors, several large bath towels, washcloth, bath blanket, cottonballs (optional), water trough or 1 1/2 yards of 60-inch-wide plastic to make a trough, electric blow dryer or curlers (optional).
2. Raise the bed to the highest horizontal position. Lower the headrest and lower the side rails on the side you are working. Position the client with his head close to the edge of the bed. Place bed protectors under his head.
3. Place a chair, with a bed protector on it, at the side of the bed with the back of the chair near the client's head. The back should be touching the mattress.

4. Inspect the client's hair for knots and/or lice. Lice are little black insects that live on the scalp and hair. If you notice any, stop the procedure and call your supervisor. Comb knots out before you start the shampoo.

5. Put a bath blanket on the client and fold the sheet and regular blanket to the bottom of the bed. If the client wishes, put cotton balls in his ears to prevent water from splashing into them. Cover the client's eyes with the washcloth.

6. Place the water trough under the client's head with the open edge in the pail on the chair.

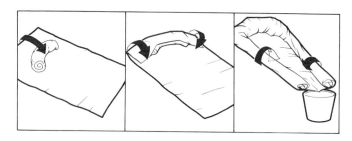

7. Pour water from the pitcher over the client's hair. Wet the whole head. Apply shampoo to the hair. Massage the hair and scalp with your fingertips, not your nails.

8. Rinse the hair thoroughly. If the client uses conditioner, apply it according to the directions on the bottle.

9. Remove the cotton balls from the client's ears. Raise the client's head and wrap it in a towel. Rub the client's hair to dry it as much as possible.

10. Remove the equipment from the bedside. Be sure the client is safe and comfortable when you leave.

11. Comb the client's hair. Style it as the client prefers. If you use a dryer, be sure it is set on cool.

12. Remove the bath blanket and replace the top sheet and regular blanket. Return the bed to its original height. Be sure the client is safe and comfortable.

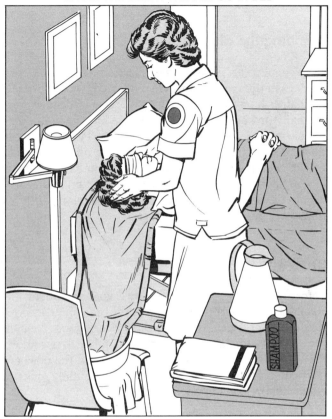

13. Clean and put away the equipment. Wash your hands.

Shampooing a Client's Hair at the Sink

This is very similar to the procedure described above except that the client is sitting or standing at the sink. Before you attempt to wash his hair, be sure the client can maintain the position at the sink. As you work observe the client continually. If the client appears to be uncomfortable or dizzy, stop immediately.

Combing the Client's Hair

If the client wears glasses, ask him to remove them. Comb and brush the hair in the style requested by the client. If the hair is long and knots easily, suggest braids. Inspect the hair for knots or lice. If there are knots, comb them out slowly and gently. If you notice lice, stop the procedure and notify your supervisor. Lice are little black insects that live on the scalp and hair. Comb each section of hair separately using a downward motion and working up toward the head. Turn the client's head gently so that you can reach the whole head.

SHAVING

Before shaving any client, be sure you have been instructed to do so. You may use a safety razor or an electric razor. *Do not use an electric razor if the client is receiving oxygen.* As you shave the client, remember to use short, firm strokes. The areas around the lips and the nose are particularly sensitive. If you should accidentally nick the client, report this to your supervisor.

Procedure: Shaving the Client's Beard

1. Assemble the equipment: basin of warm to hot water, shaving cream if using a safety razor, face towel, mirror, tissues, washcloth, after shave lotion or face powder (optional).
2. Raise the head of the bed if permitted. Raise the bed to its highest horizontal position. Lower the side rails on

the side you are working. Position the client close to the side of the bed where you are working.

3. Spread a towel under the client's chin. If he wears dentures, be sure they are in his mouth. This will make shaving easier.

4. If using a safety razor, put some warm water on the client's face or use a warm washcloth to soften the beard. Apply shaving cream generously. *Omit this step if using an electric razor.*

5. With the fingers of one hand, hold the skin taut as you shave in the direction the hair grows. Start under the sideburns and work downward over the cheeks. Work upward under the chin. Use firm, short strokes.

6. Rinse the razor in the basin often if using a safety razor.

7. Wash off the remaining shaving cream.

8. Apply after shave lotion or face powder as the client wishes.

9. Return the bed to its original position. Be sure the client is safe and comfortable.

10. Clean and put away the equipment. Wash your hands.

TOILETING

Toileting is usually an activity that is very private. The client will often have to perform this with varying amounts of assistance. Assist him in a way that is acceptable and safe to you and to the client. Often people use special words to refer to the act of elimination. If you are familiar with the words your client uses, the procedures will be easier for you both.

As you assist your client, notice the following:

- Frequency of elimination
- Color
- Odor

- Any pain with elimination
- Ability to control elimination
- Any foreign material, such as blood or mucus

There are several pieces of equipment available for use by clients who are unable to go to the bathroom.

- *Bedpan:* a receptacle into which male and female clients defecate. Female clients also use this when they urinate.
- *Urinal:* a container into which male clients urinate. There are female urinals but they are not used often.
- *Portable commode:* a chairlike piece of equipment with a pail in it. Usually this is brought directly to the bedside. The pail is emptied after each use.

Procedure: Offering the Bedpan

1. Assemble the equipment: bedpan and cover, toilet tissue, wash basin or wet washcloth, talcum powder or cornstarch, handtowel, equipment to clean the bedpan.
2. Warm the bedpan by running warm water inside it along the rim. Dry the outside and put powder or cornstarch on the part that will touch the client. This will stop his skin from sticking to the bed pan. If the client is going to move his bowels and a specimen is not needed, place several sheets of toilet paper or a slight bit of water in the bottom of the bedpan. This will make cleaning easier.
3. Raise the bed to the highest horizontal position. Lower the side rail on the side where you are standing.
4. Raise the client's gown or lower his pajamas. Keep the lower part of his body covered with the top sheet. Ask the client to bend his knees, put his feet flat on the

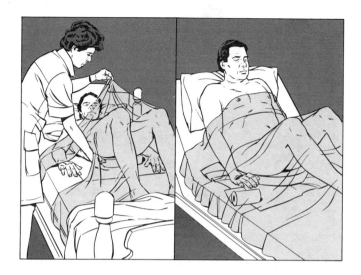

mattress and raise his hips. If necessary, slip your hand under the lower part of the client's back and help him. Place the bedpan in position with the seat of the bedpan under the buttocks and the open end toward the client's feet.

5. If the client is unable to lift his buttocks, turn him on his side with his back toward you. Put the bedpan against his buttocks and roll him over on to the bedpan.

6. Cover the client. Place the toilet tissue where the client can reach it. Provide privacy. Ask the client to signal when finished. Wash your hands if you are going to do another task.

7. Wash your hands when you return to the room. Help the client raise his hips so you can remove the bedpan and cover it immediately. If the client is unable to clean himself, it is your responsibility to do it. Turn the client on his side and clean the anal area with toilet tissue. For female clients, clean the anal area before you clean the meatus.

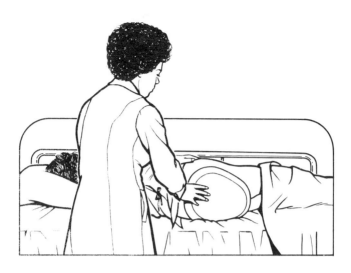

8. You may either remove the bedpan to the bathroom and return or you may put the bedpan at the side of the bed.
9. Offer the client a wet washcloth for his hands or the opportunity to wash his hands in a basin of water.
10. Return the bed to its original position. Be sure the client is safe and comfortable.
11. Measure the output if ordered. If a specimen is needed, take it. Empty the bedpan into the client's toilet. Wash the bedpan with cold water and a toilet brush if necessary. Clean and put away all the equipment. Wash your hands.

Procedure: Offering the Urinal

1. Assemble the equipment: urinal and cover, basin of water or wet washcloth, soap, towels.
2. Give the client the urinal. If he is unable to put it into place, place his penis into the opening as far as it goes.

Raise the head of the bed if the client prefers. Ask the client to signal when he is finished. If the client is unable to hold the urinal in place, you will be responsible to do this.

3. Give the client privacy. Wash your hands if you are going to do another task.

4. Wash your hands when you return to the room. Take the urinal. Cover it. You may either remove the urinal to the bathroom and return, or you may put it at the side of the bed. Offer the client a wet washcloth for his hands or the opportunity to wash his hands in a basin of water.

5. Be sure the client is safe and comfortable.

6. Measure the output if ordered. Collect a specimen if needed. Empty the urinal into the client's toilet. Wash the urinal with cold water and a toilet brush if necessary. Clean and replace all the equipment. Wash your hands.

Procedure: Assisting the Client with a Portable Commode

1. Assemble the equipment: portable bedside commode, toilet tissue, basin of water or wet washcloth, soap, towel.

2. Put the commode next to the client's bed in a safe position. Fasten the toilet paper to the commode by tying the roll to the frame with a string. You can make a holder by stretching out a coat hanger and threading the roll onto it and hooking the ends to the commode frame. Be sure to bend the ends and then tape them so they do not scratch the client. Using proper body mechanics, transfer the client to the commode.

3. If you do not have to collect a specimen or measure the output, leave a small amount of water in the bottom of the pail. This will make the cleaning easier.

4. Give the client privacy. Be sure he is safe. Wash your hands if you are going to do another task.
5. Wash your hands when you return to the client. Offer the client toilet tissue. If he is unable to clean the anal area, it is your responsibility to clean him.
6. Assist the client back to his bed.
7. Offer the client a basin of water or a wet washcloth to wash his hands.
8. Make the client comfortable.
9. Remove the pail from the commode. Cover it and carry it to the bathroom. Measure the output if ordered. Collect a specimen if it is needed. Empty the pail into the toilet, and clean it with a toilet brush. Put the pail back in the commode.
10. Wash your hands.

PERINEAL CARE

Perineal care is the gentle cleansing of the *perineal area* or *perineum*. This may be necessary following the birth of a child, surgery, or when a female client does not take a full bath but wishes to clean the genital area. This procedure promotes healing, prevents infection, and refreshes the client. When you use a squeeze bottle to direct the stream of water, you cleanse the area without damaging the skin, and you encourage the client, who cannot reach the area, to take part in the procedure.

Procedure: Care of the Perineal Area

1. Assemble the equipment: two peribottles or squeeze bottles, mild soap, clean dressings or peripads, undergarments, towels, garbage bag for soiled dressings, and warm water.

2. Remove old dressings and discard them in the paper or plastic bag. Note the color, amount, and odor of the drainage.

3. Assist the client onto the commode, toilet, or bedpan. Fill one bottle with warm soapy water and the other with warm clean water. Place the bottle filled with soapy water parallel to the perineum. Let the water drain over the perineum. Move the bottle so that the whole perineal area is cleansed. Do this for at least two minutes. You may have to refill the bottle. Rinse the perineum with the plain warm water from the second bottle.

4. Assist the client to stand up or get off the bedpan. Pat the area dry. Assist the client with clean dressings and putting on undergarments. Make the client comfortable.

5. Clean and put away the equipment. Wash your hands.

12

Rehabilitation of the Client

REHABILITATION

Rehabilitation is the process of relearning how to function, despite a disability, in the best possible way as an independent person. This may include using equipment, learning exercises or learning to use a body part in a new way. Factors taken into consideration when a rehabilitation program is formulated are

- How much active or passive motion does the client have?
- What are the client's sensory deficits in vision, hearing, touch, speech, and balance? What activity can realistically be expected? What are the client's priorities?
- What is the attitude of the client: depressed? motivated? wanting to be independent?
- What was the previous level of the client's function? If a person did not have the desire to do something before becoming disabled, he may not be motivated to do it afterward.

- What equipment does the client have? What can be obtained?
- Are there environmental barriers? Are there things in the client's home that make it difficult for him to assume his own care? Are there many stairs? Is the lighting poor? Is there only one bathroom that cannot be altered to meet his needs?
- Is there a support system composed of family and friends that will help the client when you are not there? Do they want the client to gain independence?

Working with Physical Therapists

A physical therapist is a person who, in conjunction with a physician, establishes a routine of exercises that will strengthen muscles and assist with purposeful motion.

- Do not start any exercise regime until you have been specifically instructed to do so.
- Never take a client beyond the point of pain. Report client pain to your supervisor. Do not force a body part into a position it will not go easily.
- Report if the client does not or cannot do the exercises when you are not in the house. Include the family as you exercise the client.
- Use the flat part of your hand to grasp the body part in a slow, steady movement.
- Talk to the client as you exercise with him. Explain what you are doing and why even if it appears the client does not understand your words. The tone of your voice is understood.
- Follow a logical sequence, such as starting at the head and working toward the feet. Follow that sequence each time the exercises are done.

Range-of-Motion

Range of motion exercises take the client through all possible motion of the joint. Do not change the exercise plan unless you have been told to do so. There are four types of range-of-motion exercises:

- *Passive:* The client does not help.
- *Active/assist:* The client actively moves the body part and the helper moves it slightly farther than the client can.
- *Active:* The client does the entire exercise.
- *Resistive:* The client actively moves the body part and the helper provides resistance so that the muscle works harder. Resistance can be provided by hand or by using weights.

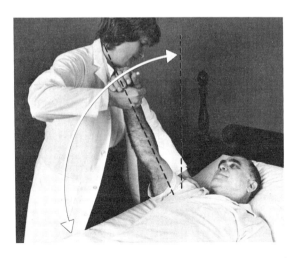

Shoulder Flexion: With elbows straight, raise arm over head, then lower, *keeping arm in front of you* the whole time.

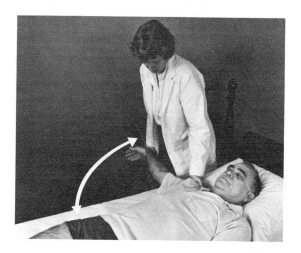

Shoulder Abduction and Adduction: With elbows straight, raise arm over head, then lower, *keeping arm out to the side* the whole time.

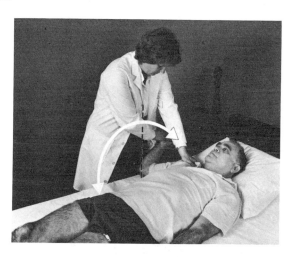

Shoulder Internal & External Rotation: Bring arm out to the side. Do NOT bring elbow out to shoulder level. Turn arm back and forth so forearm points down toward feet, then up toward head. With arm alongside body and elbow bent at 90°, turn arm so forearm points across stomach, then out to the side.

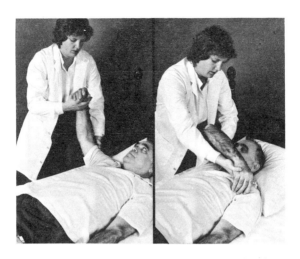

Shoulder Horizontal Abduction and Adduction: *Keeping arm at shoulder level*, reach across chest past opposite shoulder, then reach out to the side.

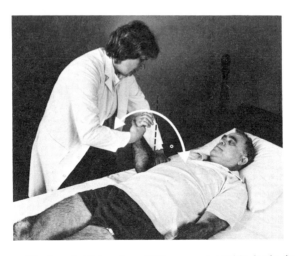

Elbow Flexion & Extension: With arm alongside body, bend elbow to touch shoulder, then straighten elbow out again.

160

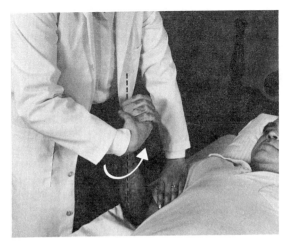

Forearm Pronation & Supination: With arm alongside the body and elbow bent to 90° (a right angle), turn forearm so palm faces first toward head, then toward feet.

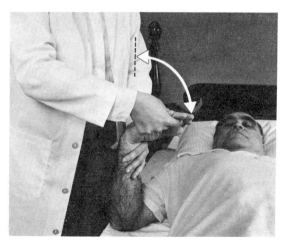

Wrist Flexion & Extension: Bend wrist up and down.

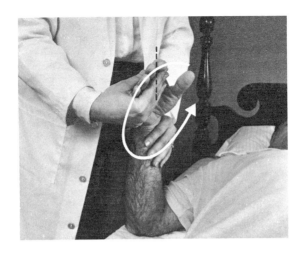

Wrist Flexion & Extension: Bend wrist back and forth, and in a circle.

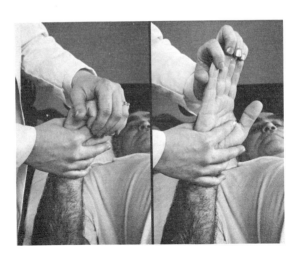

Finger Flexion & Extension: Make a fist, then straighten fingers out together.

162

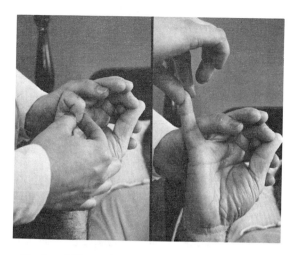

Finger Flexion & Extension: Touch tip of each finger to its base, then straighten each finger in turn.

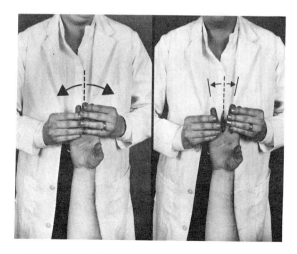

Finger Adduction & Abduction: With fingers straight, squeeze fingers together, then spread them apart.

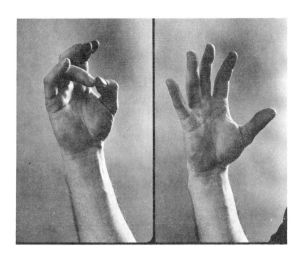

Finger/Thumb Opposition: Touch thumb to the tip of each finger to make a circle. Open hand fully between touching each finger.

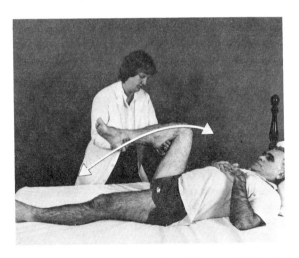

Hip/Knee Flexion & Extension: Bend Knee and bring it up toward chest, keeping foot off bed. Lower leg to bed, straightening knee as it goes down.

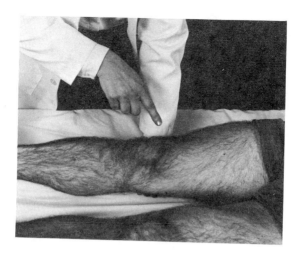

Quad Sets: With leg flat on bed, tighten thigh muscles to straighten the knee, *hard*, pushing it into the bed. Hold for a count of 5, then relax. Repeat exercise with rolled towel under the knee.

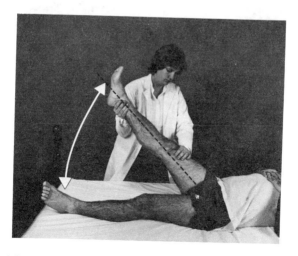

Straight Leg Raising: Keeping the knee straight, raise leg up off the bed. Return slowly to the bed, keeping the knee straight.

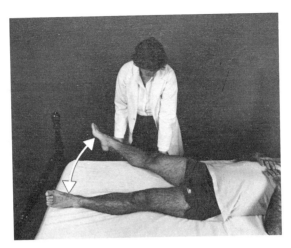

Hip Abduction & Adduction: With leg flat on bed and knee kept pointing to ceiling, slide leg out to the side. Then slide it back to touch across the other leg.

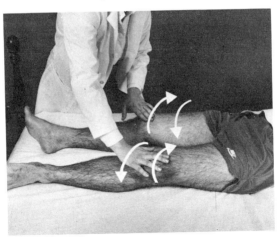

Hip Internal & External Rotation: With legs flat on bed and feet apart, turn both legs so knees face outward. Then turn them in so knees face each other.

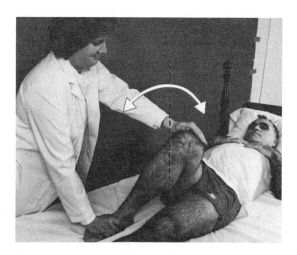

Hip Internal & External Rotation (Variation): With one knee bent and foot flat on the bed, turn leg so knee moves out to the side, then inward across the other leg. Do each leg separately.

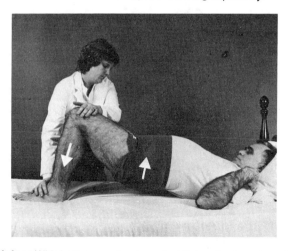

Bridging: With both knees bent up, feet flat on bed, push on bed with feet to raise hips (as in lifting for a bedpan). Hold for a count of 5, then relax.

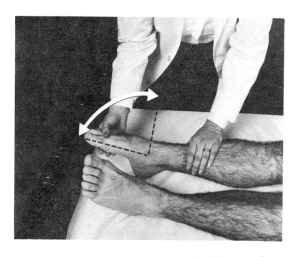

Ankle Dorsiflexion & Extension: Bend ankles up, down, and from side to side.

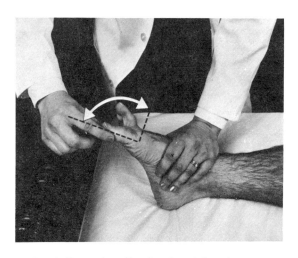

Toe Flexion & Extension: Bend and straighten toes.

168

Choosing a Chair for the Client

- The chair should provide good support to the client's back.
- The type of chair that provides the client the most safety and independence is the best chair.
- The client must be able to get out of the chair easily and safely.
- What types of chairs are available?
- Does the chair have arms? Can the client rest his feet on the floor?

Transferring a Client

- Know your capabilities. Can you assist this client? Can the client help you? Do you need a piece of equipment to help make the transfer safe? Do you need another person to help?
- Concentrate on what you are doing. Do not talk to another person when you are transferring the client. Be alert to changes in the client such as dizzy spells, weakness, or lapses in his concentration.
- Keep your directions short and simple.
- Use the same sequence of directions each time you transfer a client.

Procedure: Helping a Client to Sit up in Bed

1. Roll the client on his side, facing you. Bend his knees. Reach one arm over to hold him back of his knees. Position your other arm under the neck and shoulder area.
2. Position your feet with a wide base of support and your center of gravity close to the bed. On the count of "one, two, three" shift your weight to your back leg while swinging the client's legs over the edge of the

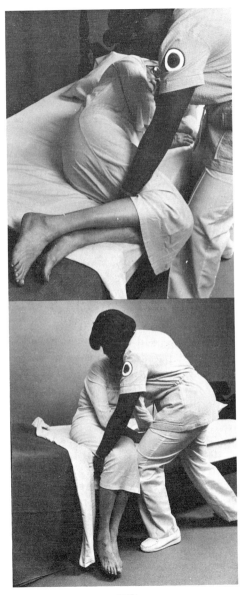

bed and pulling his shoulders, bringing the client to a sitting position.

3. Remain in front of the client keeping both hands on him for support until he is stable. Proceed with the rest of the transfer, or let the client remain in this position.

Procedure: Using a Portable Mechanical Client Lift

1. Assemble the equipment: mechanical lift, sling, chair.

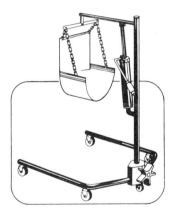

2. Position the chair next to the bed with the back of the chair in line with the headboard. Slide the sling under the client in the correct place.

3. Attach the sling to the mechanical lift. The hooks should be in place through the metal, which should face outward.

4. Have the client fold both arms across his chest. This prevents injury and assists with balance.

5. Using the crank, lift the client off the bed. Guide the client's legs. Swing the client over the chair and lower him slowly. Talk to the client during this procedure.

6. Remove the hooks from the frame. If possible, leave the sling in place. Be sure the client is safe and comfortable in the chair.
7. To put the client back into bed, reverse the procedure.

Procedure: Helping a Client to Stand

1. If the client is in bed, he must get to a sitting position at the edge of the bed. If he is in a chair, he must move to the edge of his seat. Put on the client's slippers or shoes.
2. "Move to the front of your chair or bed. Put your hands on the arms of the chair or the mattress." Place one of your knees between the client's knees. If the client has a weak knee, brace it with your knee.
3. "Put the strongest foot under you on the floor." Bend your knees and lean onto your forward foot to place

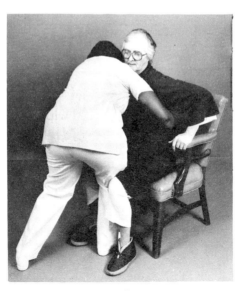

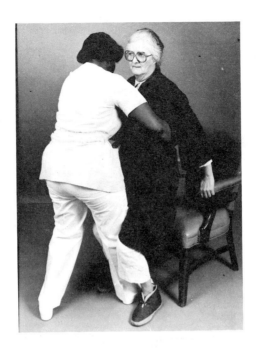

the same side arm around the client's waist. Place your other hand at the other side of the client's waist. You have now encircled the client, and are holding him at his center of gravity.

4. "On the count of three, push down with your arms, lean forward and stand up." Hold the client tightly. On the count of three, rock your weight to your back foot.

Procedure: Helping a Client to Sit from a Standing Position

1. Perform the procedure described above in reverse.
2. Be sure the client can feel the chair or bed with the back of his legs. Direct the client to reach back for the arms

of the chair or the mattress of the bed. Direct the activity so the client does not fall.

Procedure: Pivot Transfer
from the Bed to Chair

1. Place the wheelchair or chair at a 45 degree angle to the bed. Be sure the wheels are locked and the chair is secure.
2. Bring the client to a sitting position at the edge of the bed. Put slippers or shoes on his feet. Explain the procedure to the client.
   a. He will come to a standing position.
   b. He will reach for the arm of the chair, pivot and sit.
   c. You will keep your foot near the client's foot for extra support.

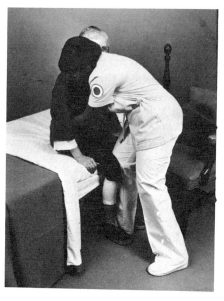

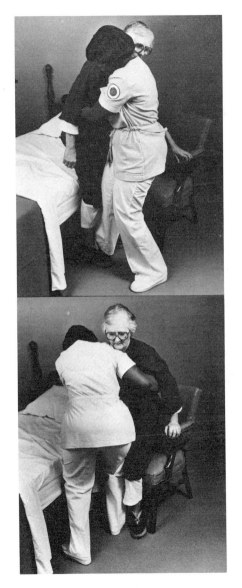

3. You will use good body mechanics to support and guide him during the whole procedure.
4. Secure the client in the chair. Be sure he is safe and comfortable. Wash your hands.

Procedure: Pivot Transfer from Chair to Bed

1. Perform the procedure described above.
2. Direct the client to come to a standing position.
3. Direct the client to reach for the bed and pivot. Help and guide him.
4. Direct the activity so the client does not fall.
5. Make sure the client is safe and comfortable.
6. Put away the chair. Wash your hands.

Ambulation Activities and Assistive Walking Devices

As the client gains strength, you may remain with him for directions and in case you are needed. You may not have to actually touch the client or give physical support. Encourage the client to do as much for himself as he safely can, but do not leave him alone until you are certain he is safe. As you provide minimal assistance, remember

- Stand on the weaker side.
- Use a guarding belt for extra support if needed. One hand should be on the guarding belt, the other hand in front of the collarbone on the weaker side.
- Always apply basic body mechanics when using an assistive device. Be sure the client can safely use the device and that you are familiar with it.
- Use the same procedure each time the client uses the device. This way, you will set up a routine.

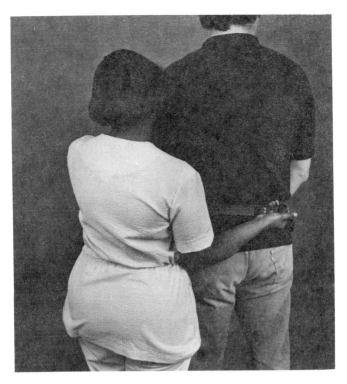

Canes, crutches, and walkers are pieces of assistive equipment. Each one is prescribed by a physical therapist and fitted to the needs, size, and capabilities of the client. All equipment is used after the client has come to a standing position. The cane is used on the client's stronger side. By doing this, the base of support is widened between the cane and the client's weaker side. A walker is used to give extra support. It will provide support only when all four legs are on the ground. If the walker is being moved, the client should be standing still and the walker should be picked up and moved, not slid along the ground.

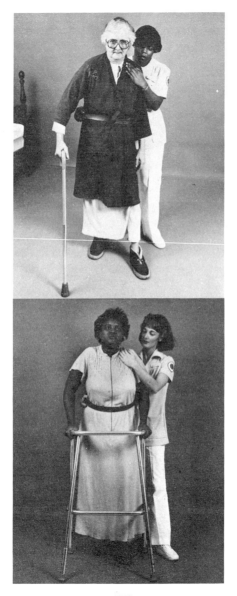

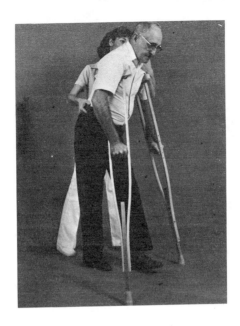

SPEECH AND LANGUAGE THERAPY

The *speech-language pathologist* is the professional who evaluates the need for speech therapy and plans the therapy in conjunction with the physician. A client may need speech and language therapy if he has a disorder that affects parts of his brain, lips, tongue, or throat.

Aphasia

Injury to the brain may cause a loss of speech or language ability which is called *aphasia.* Usually the injury is from a cerebrovascular accident or CVA or stroke. A *cerebrovascular accident* means that a blood clot, hemorrhage, or vascular spasm in the brain has stopped oxygen from reaching the part of the brain tissue causing it to stop functioning. Damage to brain tissue may also be caused by a blow to the head or a tumor.

An aphasic person may have difficulty in all areas of communication. It may be hard for him to read, write, speak, or understand. Aphasia does not mean that the person is unable to think. It only means he is unable to communicate. The kind of aphasia is determined by the area of the brain that was injured.

Expressive aphasia means the client has difficulty expressing thoughts and sometimes writing. The client always has the feeling of having the words right on the tip of his tongue, as though he is about to say something and then suddenly forgets.

Receptive aphasia means that the client has difficulty receiving or understanding what is heard. It is as though the client is hearing a foreign language and does not have any means of making himself understood. This person may have

- No interest in watching television or listening to the radio
- No interest in reading
- No ability to follow directions
- No ability to answer questions appropriately

The behavior of an aphasic person may seem rude. Remember that the person is an intelligent adult who simply cannot communicate easily. Such an individual will be most cooperative and less frustrated when you treat him like an adult. A client with aphasia

- Tires easily
- Laughs or cries frequently without apparent reason
- Uses profanity without meaning to do so
- Repeats the same words over and over

The speech pathologist will prescribe speech exercises. Do not change them unless you have been told to do so. Exercises may include the use of pictures, the printed word, and/or facial strengthening exercises. You will also be asked to observe and report how the client makes his needs known, how he responds to the therapy, and how the family interacts with the client.

When communicating with a person with aphasia, do

- Get the attention of the client before you speak to him.
- Speak slowly. Keep instructions simple. Keep the conversation about the client's immediate needs.
- Ask questions that have simple yes or no answers.
- Encourage the client to use common expressions, such as "hello" and "good-bye."
- Give the client time to reply after asking a question,
- Give the client an opportunity to listen to the television, radio, and family conversation.
- Meals and dressing times are good opportunities to encourage the client to speak. Let him ask for what he needs. The aphasic client may say a word correctly sometimes and sometimes may forget it. Making the effort is the important thing.
- Show the client understanding, not pity. By your body language you indicate patience and acceptance or impatience and frustration.
- If the client cannot express himself, or if you cannot understand him say, "Let's forget it now and come back to it later. The words will probably come when you are not trying so hard."
- As you care for the client, tell him what you are doing and refer to his body parts by name.

When communicating with an aphasic client don't

- Answer for the client, finish his sentences, or interrupt him if he is capable of speaking.
- Confuse the client with too much chatter or too many people talking at once.
- Discuss the client's emotional reactions and problems in his presence.
- Embarrass the client or treat him like a baby. If he does not understand you, do not shout. Simply rephrase your words.

Dealing with a Hearing Loss

Some people are born with a hearing loss. Some people lose their hearing due to an accident, drug reaction, or deterioration of the nerves. The person who is hard of hearing may feel that others are mumbling; he may avoid social activities because he cannot take part in them. He may become frustrated and angry.

Hearing Aids

The hearing aid earmold is custom made to fit the ear. If it does not fit snugly there will be a high pitched whistling noise when the aid is turned on. If the earmold is dirty, or if ear wax is clogging it, sound will not pass through. The earmold should be wiped clean with a tissue after each wearing. Clean the earmold with soap and water. Follow the directions that the manufacturer gives. Do not use alcohol or cleaning fluid.

- Keep the hearing aid away from heat such as hair dryers.
- Do not get the hearing aid wet.
- Do not spray the hearing aid with hair spray.
- Do not twist the wires.

When putting the batteries into the earmold, match the "+" on the battery to the "+" on the earmold. A battery lasts about ten days. You can remove the battery from the earmold when it is not in use. Store unused batteries in a cool, dry place. If the hearing aid does not work, check to see if

- The battery is put in correctly.
- The aid is turned on and the volume is loud enough.
- The earmold is clean.

When talking to a hearing impaired person:

- Get his attention before you start speaking.
- Talk face to face. Your client will understand more if he can see your face.
- Do not chew food or gum when you are speaking.
- Do not exaggerate your words. Speak at a normal rate of speed.

WORKING WITH OCCUPATIONAL THERAPISTS

Many clients are unable to perform useful actions with a specific body part. This is called *functional limitation*. A client with this type of limitation needs assistance with *activities of daily living*. Many *adaptive pieces* of equipment exist. The occupational therapist of the local surgical supply store can be of help in deciding which piece of equipment is most appropriate for the client. Often this equipment must be purchased by the client. Therefore, consult an expert *before* the purchase is made.

The occupational therapist focuses on increasing the functional ability of the client within his environment. This increases the client's self esteem and ability to take part in the normal functions of the family. As the occupational therapist works with the client, routines and exercises are established. Follow these routines so that the client does not get confused. Be sure that you are familiar with the pieces of equipment and how you are to assist the client to use them.

- If the client says, "I can't," assist him with the routine. Perhaps you will each do part of it.
- If the client shows signs of pain or being tired, stop.
- Be observant for changes in the client's ability and function. Point out positive changes in the client's ability.

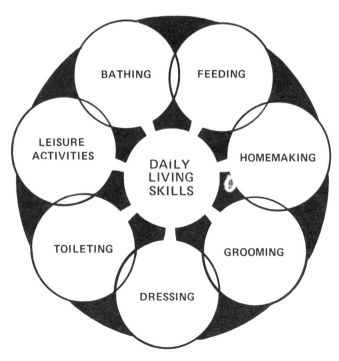

- Do not attempt any technique you have not been shown.
- As the client's abilities increase and change, change your role accordingly. Remember, the goal is to help the client become as independent and safe as possible in his home.
- Does the client need a piece of equipment to help?

TOILETING

Since toileting is a very basic and usually private task, assist the client with this procedure only as much as necessary. Tell the client what part of the procedure you will do and what part he will do.

Toileting in Bed

- Provide a *pulling braid*, which is made by braiding three 4-inch wide strips of torn sheeting lengthwise and tying the braid to the bed frame. The other end is knotted. This can be very helpful when a client wants to sit up or change position.
- Provide for privacy.
- Do not take the client out of bed unless you have been instructed to do so.

Toileting on a Commode

- Be sure the commode is standing securely.
- Place the commode in the position in which the client was instructed to use it. Assist with the transfer as necessary.
- Fasten the toilet paper to the commode in a convenient place for the client. Tie the roll with a string or make a holder out of a coat hanger. Bend the ends and tape them to avoid scratching the client. Place the roll on the client's strongest side.

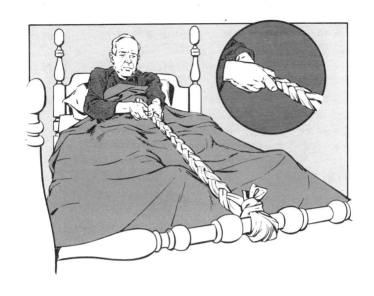

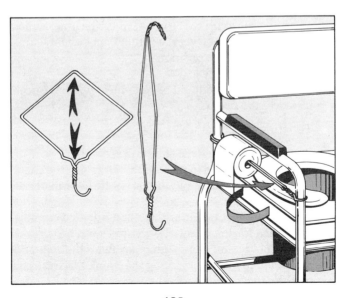

- Offer the client a washcloth to clean his genitalia and/or his hands.
- Provide for privacy.

Toileting in the Bathroom

If the client uses the toilet, you may suggest the use of a frame around the commode. A frame provides additional support. Hang an 8- by 10-inch piece of plastic between the back of the frame and the commode so that the plastic hangs into the toilet. This prevents splashing of urine. Be sure to rinse the plastic off after each use.

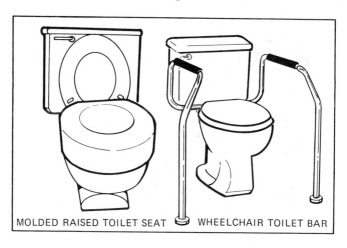

MOLDED RAISED TOILET SEAT   WHEELCHAIR TOILET BAR

BATHING

Bathing stimulates the body, increases circulation, increases muscle and joint movement, and encourages the client to become aware of his body. It may also trigger feelings and experiences the client had before his disability. The occupational therapist will show the client how to bathe in as independent a manner as possible. This will be done by adapting the usual procedure to meet the client's needs and by using adaptive equipment. This procedure will probably take longer than if you bathed the client yourself. Remember that your role, however, is to teach the client to be independent and function when you are not there. So, take your time and allow the client to do the same.

- Use the equipment as you have been instructed. Do not change the routine unless you check with the therapist.
- Thin washcloths and thin towels are easier for the client to use.
- Wash the involved side first. Remind the client to wash in places he may not feel or he may forget. By placing a mirror near him, the client can see where the soap is on his body.
- Stabilize the soap on a washcloth, soap dish, or rubber disk.
- Drape a well-soaped washcloth over the palm of the involved hand while resting on the client's lap. Then he can lean forward and cradle his uninvolved arm in the hand and slide it back and forth to wash it.
- Drape a towel in his involved hand and rub the uninvolved hand over them. This way the client can wash and dry both hands independently.
- Do not put the client into a tub or shower until you have been instructed to do so.

DRESSING AND GROOMING

Encourage the client to dress in street clothes even if he is wheelchair bound or bedbound. Getting dressed affects not only the client's sense of well-being, but influences the way in which others react to him. Dressing allows the client to use his limbs, his coordination, and his balance. With certain limitations, clients find some pieces of clothing to be difficult to put on. However, most types of clothing can be altered or redesigned not only to allow the client to wear them, but also to put them on without any help.

- Always dress the weak or involved side first.
- Allow the client to select his own clothing. Encourage him to select clothes that are roomy, that will stretch, or that have wide openings. These are easier to put on and take off.
- Encourage the client to wear soft fabrics that do not itch or irritate the skin.
- Lay out the client's clothes in the order he will put them on. Always use the same order and the same routine.
- Encourage the client to take care of his clothes. He can fold them and stack them in a drawer. This can be done both after wearing and after the clothes are washed.
- Rearrange drawers so that they are accessible to the client.

MEALS

Supervise the client in the kitchen. Use the devices the occupational therapist demonstrates. Encourage the client to take an active part in meal preparation if that is a usual activity.

- Use a cutting board to prepare vegetables.
- Use small containers that are easy to pick up.
- Prepare food that the client can easily and safely eat.
- Cut the food and prepare it as he prefers. Use plastic containers and plates rather than glass. Use the uten-

sils that have large handles, mitts to hold the utensils, and guards for the plates to prevent food from being pushed off the plate. These may have to be specially purchased.

Be sure the client can swallow the food and the liquid. Be sure he can safely bring the utensil to his face. Often a shaving mirror placed in front of the client will give him visual clues as to where the utensils are and where his mouth is.

Encourage the client and his family to eat together. Often the client will prefer to eat alone since he may be slower than the rest of the family and he may spill or drop his food. Protect the client's clothes but do not treat him like a baby. Eating is a social time for most families and the client will benefit from the socialization.

LEISURE ACTIVITIES

Pleasant activities and those that pass the time are very important. You may play cards, do crossword puzzles, or play games with the client. These are therapeutic activities. These activities expand the ability of the client and increase his sense of well-being. They also help with muscle coordination and the thinking process. There are many adapted games, cards, and activities that can be specially purchased.

13

Measuring and Recording Vital Signs

VITAL SIGNS

The term *vital signs* refers to body temperature, pulse rate, respiratory rate, and blood pressure. When the body is not functioning normally, the measurable rates of vital signs change.

- Be sure your equipment is in good working order.
- Be sure your handwriting is clear and easy to read.
- Do not guess if you are unsure of a reading.
- Write down the readings immediately after you take them.

The decision to check vital signs is based upon the client's present condition, his past history, and his prognosis. You will also be told when to report the readings. If you are in doubt about reporting a reading immediately or just writing it down, report it.

Vital signs should be checked and reported

- according to the schedule you have been assigned

- if you notice a change in the client's condition
- after a fall

There are many charts showing the "normal" readings for temperature, respirations, pulse, and blood pressure. Although these are good guides, it is better to compare these with the client's usual readings, since each of us has a slightly different "normal" reading.

If a client asks you what his vital signs are, you should tell him. It is his body and he has a right to know how it is functioning. There are clients who do not wish to know this information. Do not force them. Respect their wishes. There are also times when you will be asked not to tell the client his vital signs. Abide by the wishes of the physician and the family even if you do not always agree with them.

Measuring Body Temperature

Body temperature is a measurement of the amount of heat in the body. The balance between the heat produced and the heat lost is body temperature. Normal ranges of body temperature are

Oral: 97.6° to 99°F (36.4° to 37.2°C)

Rectal: 98.6° to 100°F (37° to 37.8°C)

Axillary: 96.6° to 98°F (35.9° to 36.7°C)

Symbols used in recording temperature are:

°	degrees	R	rectal temperature
F	Fahrenheit	O	oral temperature
C	Centigrade	A	Axillary temperature

When recording a temperature, indicate the reading and how it was taken.

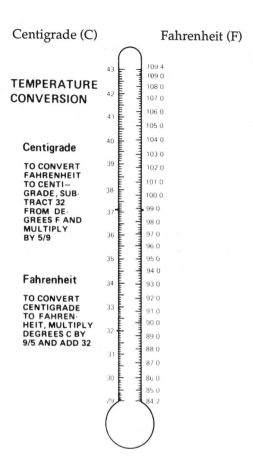

Centigrade (C)   Fahrenheit (F)

**TEMPERATURE
CONVERSION**

Centigrade

TO CONVERT
FAHRENHEIT
TO CENTI—
GRADE, SUB-
TRACT 32
FROM DE-
GREES F AND
MULTIPLY
BY 5/9

Fahrenheit

TO CONVERT
CENTIGRADE
TO FAHREN-
HEIT, MULTIPLY
DEGREES C BY
9/5 AND ADD 32

Types of Thermometers

All thermometers have a way of indicating temperature. Glass thermometers, the most common type, are
hollow tubes with mercury inside. The bulb end is the
part inserted into the client. When the bulb is heated, the
mercury rises. The place it stops rising indicates the
temperature. Digital thermometers and paper indicating
strips work differently.

Oral: used to measure temperature by mouth and to obtain the axillary temperature. The bulb is long and thin.

Rectal: used to measure temperature by inserting the bulb into the rectum. The bulb is small and round.

Security: used to take an infant's temperature but can also be used for adults. It is very strong. Usually, the thermometers with the red knob are used for rectal temperatures and those with green knobs for oral ones.

Safety Considerations

- Do not expect a client to talk with a thermometer in his mouth. If the client must talk or sneeze, remove the thermometer.
- Handle thermometers carefully. The liquid inside (mercury) is a poison when it comes in contact with the skin. Prevent breaking or chipping of the thermometer.
- Keep the thermometer in its case, not loose in a drawer.
- Do not clean a thermometer with hot water. Use cold water, soap and friction.

Procedure: Shaking Down a Thermometer

1. Assemble the equipment: a thermometer in a container.
2. Check that there are no cracks or chips in the thermometer. Hold it firmly between your fingers and your thumb at the stem end.
3. Stand clear of any hard surfaces. Shake your hand loosely from the wrist as if you were shaking water from your hands. Do this several times until the mercury is at the lowest point.

4. Always shake a thermometer before and after use. Clean and put away the equipment.

Procedure: Reading a Fahrenheit Thermometer

1. With your thumb and first two fingers, hold the thermometer by the stem at eye level. Turn the thermometer back and forth between your fingers until you can clearly see the column of mercury.
2. Notice the scale or calibrations. Each long line stands for one degree. Each of the short lines stands for two-tenths (0.2) of a degree.
3. Between the long lines that represent 98° and 99°F, look for a longer line with an arrow directly beneath it. This points to the normal body temperature of 98.6°F. Look at the end of the mercury column. Notice the line or number where the mercury ends. If it is on one of the short lines, notice the previous long line toward the bulb. The temperature reading is the degree marked by the long line plus two, four, six, and so forth tenths of a degree. For example, if the mercury ends after the 99 line on the second short line, the temperature is 99.4°F. If the mercury ends between two lines, use the closest line.
4. Write down the client's temperature as soon as you can. If you don't, you will forget it. Follow the format used by your agency.

Procedure: Reading a Centigrade (Celsius) Thermometer

1. With your thumb and first two fingers, hold the thermometer by the stem at eye level. Turn the thermom-

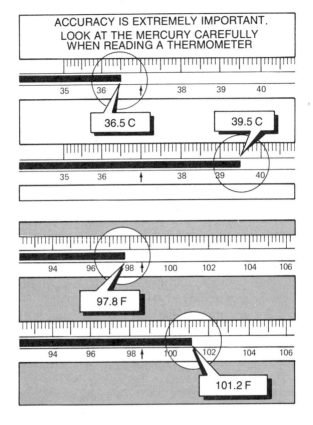

ACCURACY IS EXTREMELY IMPORTANT.
LOOK AT THE MERCURY CAREFULLY
WHEN READING A THERMOMETER

36.5 C

39.5 C

97.8 F

101.2 F

eter back and forth between your fingers until you can clearly see the column of mercury.

2. Notice the scale or calibrations. Each long line stands for one degree. Each of the short lines stands for one-tenth (0.1) of a degree. Look at the end of the mercury column. Notice the line or number where the mercury ends. If it is one of the short lines, notice the previous long line toward the bulb. If the mercury ends after the long line marked 36 and on the third short line after it, the temperature is 36.3 °C. If the mercury ends after the

long line marked 37 and on the eighth short line, the reading is 37.8°C.

3. Write down the client's temperature as soon as you can. If you don't, you will forget it. Follow the format used by your agency.

Procedure: Cleaning a Thermometer

1. Assemble the equipment: thermometer, tissue and/or cotton balls, soap, cool running water.
2. Holding the thermometer at the stem, wipe the thermometer off from the stem to the bulb. Throw away the tissue.
3. Soap a tissue. Rotate the soapy tissue around the thermometer from the stem to the bulb. Holding the thermometer under cool running water, repeat the process. Discard the tissue.

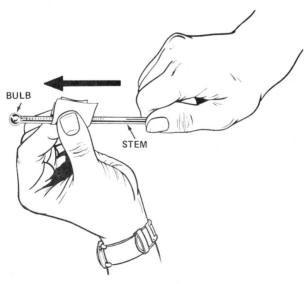

BULB

STEM

4. Dry the thermometer with a tissue. Put the thermometer away in its case.

Procedure: Measuring an Oral Temperature

Be sure the client can safely close his mouth around the thermometer. If he cannot, do not put the thermometer in his mouth.

1. Assemble the equipment: clean oral thermometer in a case, tissue or paper towel, pad and pencil, watch.
2. If the client has recently had a hot or cold drink or he has smoked, wait ten minutes before taking his temperature.
3. When you are sure there are no cracks or chips on the thermometer, shake it down until the mercury is below the calibrations. Run the thermometer under cool water. This will make it more pleasant in the client's mouth.
4. Ask the client to lift up his tongue. Place the bulb end of the thermometer under his tongue. Ask the client to keep his lips closed gently around the thermometer without biting it. Stay with the client if you feel he will not keep his mouth closed.
5. Leave the thermometer in place for eight minutes. (If the policy of your agency is to leave the thermometer in place for a different length of time, follow your policy.)
6. Take the thermometer out of the client's mouth. Hold the stem end and wipe the thermometer with a tissue from the stem end to the bulb. Discard the tissue and read the temperature.
7. Record the temperature. Shake down the thermometer.

INSERTING THE ORAL THERMOMETER

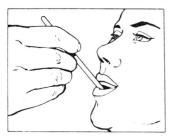

A. Insert the thermometer gently into the client's mouth under the tongue.

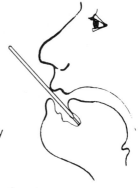

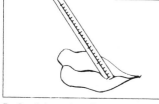

B. Position the thermometer to the side of the mouth.

C. Instruct the client to keep the thermometer under the tongue by gently closing the lips around the thermometer.

Measuring Rectal Temperature

A rectal temperature is taken when the physician specifically orders it and when the client is

- An infant or child or cannot safely use an oral thermometer
- Having warm or cold applications to his face or neck
- Finding it hard to breathe through his nose
- Suffering from dry or inflamed mouth
- Confused, unconscious, delirious, or restless
- Receiving continuous oxygen
- Recovering from major surgery in the area of his face or neck

- Partially paralyzed, as from a stroke, and cannot close his mouth or hold the thermometer

Procedure: Measuring a Rectal Temperature

1. Assemble the equipment: rectal thermometer in a case, tissues, lubricating jelly, pad and pencil, a watch.
2. Lower the back rest of the bed. Ask the client to turn on his side. If he is unable to do this, position him safely so that his buttocks are exposed.
3. Take the thermometer out of the case. When you are sure there are no cracks or chips on the thermometer, shake it down below the calibrations.
4. Put a small amount of lubricating jelly on a piece of tissue. Lubricate the bulb of the thermometer.
5. With one hand, raise the upper buttock until you see the anus. With the other hand, gently insert the thermometer 1 inch through the anus into the rectum.

    If the client is an infant, remove the diaper and lay the baby on his back. Raise his legs with one hand and insert the thermometer with the other half an inch into the rectum. Hold the thermometer while it is in the child's rectum.

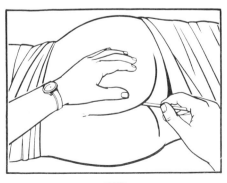

6. Hold the thermometer in place for three minutes if you have any doubt that the client will remain still.

7. Remove the thermometer from the rectum. Holding the stem, wipe it with a tissue from the stem to the bulb. Discard the tissue and read the temperature. Record the reading. Note this is a rectal temperature by writing "R" next to the numbers.

Procedure: Measuring an Axillary Temperature

1. Assemble your equipment: oral thermometer in a container, tissue, pad and pencil, a watch.

2. Take the thermometer out of the case. Inspect it for cracks. If you find any, do not use the thermometer. Shake down the thermometer until the mercury is below the calibrations.

3. Remove the client's arm from the shirt or blouse sleeve. If the axillary area is wet, pat it dry.

4. Place the bulb of the thermometer in the center of the armpit in an upright position. Put the client's arm across his chest to hold the thermometer securely in place. Hold it in place if you feel the client is too weak or cannot do it. Leave the thermometer in place for ten minutes.

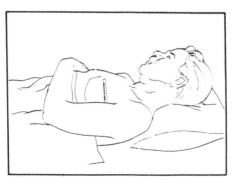

5. Remove the thermometer. Holding the stem, wipe it with a tissue from the stem to the bulb. Read the temperature. Record the reading. Note this is an axillary temperature by writing "A" next to the numbers.

Using a Plastic Sheath over a Thermometer

Plastic sheaths are used to protect the thermometer from the client's secretions and to aid in the cleaning of the thermometer. The use of the sheath does not mean you may skip the washing of the thermometer. Sheaths for rectal and oral thermometers are different. Directions for using sheaths come with them.

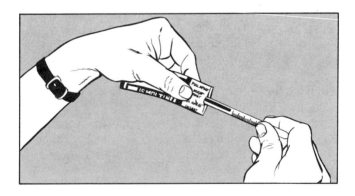

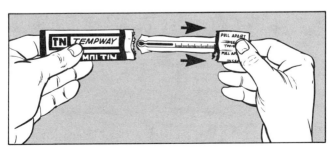

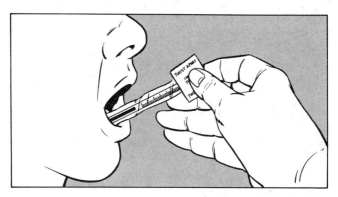

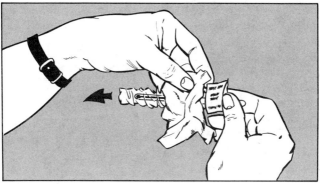

Measuring the Pulse Rate

Each time the heart beats, it pumps a certain amount of blood into the arteries. This causes the arteries to expand. Between heartbeats, the arteries contract and return to normal size. The heart pumps the blood in a steady rhythm. The rhythmic expansion and contraction of the arteries, which can be measured to show how fast the heart is beating, is called the *pulse*.

At certain places on the body, the pulse can be felt easily under a person's fingers. One of the easiest places

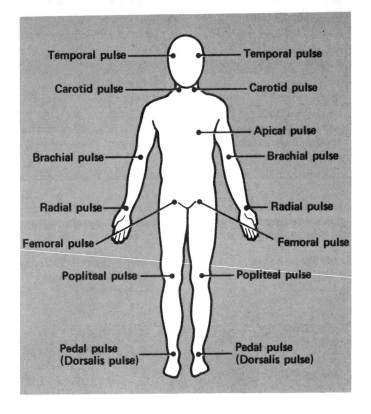

to feel the pulse is at the wrist. This is called the *radial pulse* because you are feeling the radial artery. The *apical pulse* is the pulse measured at the apex of the heart. You will use a *stethoscope* to measure this. You may use one with a *bell* or a flat, round end called a *diaphragm*.

The *apical-radial deficit* is the difference between the count you hear as you take the apical pulse and the count you feel as you take the radial pulse.

When taking a pulse, you must be able to report accurately the following:

- *Rate:* the number of beats per minute

- *Rhythm:* the regularity of the pulse beats, that is, whether the length of time between beats is steady and regular
- *Force:* whether it is bounding or weak

NORMAL PULSE RATES (PER MINUTE) FOR DIFFERENT AGE GROUPS

BEFORE BIRTH	140-150
AT BIRTH	130-140
FIRST YEAR	115-130
CHILDHOOD YEARS	80-115
ADULT YEARS	72-80
LATER YEARS	60-72

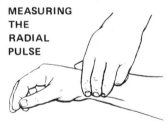

MEASURING THE RADIAL PULSE

Procedure: Measuring the Radial Pulse

1. Assemble the equipment: watch with a second hand, pad and pencil.
2. Ask the client to sit or lie down. The client's hand should be well supported and resting comfortably.
3. Place the tips of your middle three fingers on the palm side of the client's wrist in line with his thumb next to the bone. Press lightly until you feel the beat. (If you press too hard, you will stop the flow of blood and not

feel anything. Never use your thumb since the thumb has a pulse of its own.) When you have found the pulse, note the rhythm. Note if the beat is steady or irregular. Note the force of the beat.

4. Look at the position of the second hand of your watch. Start counting the pulse beats until the second hand comes back to the same position on the clock.
   a. Method A: Count the pulse beats for one full minute. This is always done if the beat is irregular.
   b. Method B: Count the beat for 30 seconds and multiply by two.
5. Record the pulse, rate, rhythm, and force immediately.

Procedure: Measuring the Apical Pulse

1. Assemble the equipment: stethoscope and antiseptic swabs, watch with a second hand, pad and pencil.
2. Ask the client to sit or lie down.
3. Clean the ear pieces of the stethoscope with antiseptic swabs. Put the ear pieces in your ears facing forward. Warm the bell or diaphragm by holding it tightly for a few seconds.
4. Uncover the left side of the client's chest. Locate the apex of the heart by placing the stethoscope over the left breast. You should hear the heart beating loudly. Look at the position of the second hand of your watch. Start counting the pulse beats until the second hand comes back to the same position on the clock. Count the heart sounds for a full minute.
5. Record the pulse, the rhythm, and the force of the sounds.

Procedure: Measuring the Apical-Radial Deficit

1. Assemble the equipment: stethoscope, antiseptic swabs, watch with a second hand, pad and pencil.
2. Ask the client to sit or lie down.
3. Clean the ear pieces of the stethoscope with antiseptic swabs. Put the ear pieces in your ears facing forward. Warm the bell or diaphragm by holding it tightly for a few seconds.
4. There are two methods for taking the apical-radial deficit:
   a. Method A: Two people do this procedure at the same time. One counts the apical pulse for a full minute and one counts the radial pulse for a full minute. The difference between the two counts is the deficit.

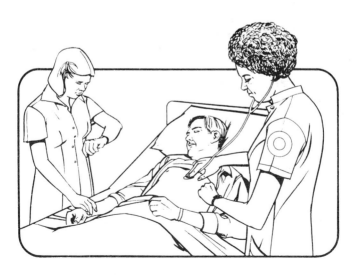

b. Method B: One person counts the apical pulse and then counts the radial pulse. The difference between the two is the deficit

5. Uncover the left side of the client's chest. Locate the apex of the heart by placing the stethoscope over the left breast. You should hear the heart beating loudly. Count the heart sounds for a full minute.

6. Record both pulses, the rhythm, and the force of the sounds for both the apical and the radial pulse.

Measuring Respirations

Respiration is the process of inhaling air and removing the waste products with exhalation. When a person breathes in, his chest expands. When he breathes out, his chest contracts. When you count respirations, watch the chest rise and fall without the client knowing it. If the client knows you are watching him breathe, he may change his breathing pattern. Besides counting respirations, notice whether the client seems to breathe easily or seems to be working hard to breathe. The latter is called *labored respirations*.

Normally adults breathe at a rate from 10 to 20 times a minute. Children breathe more rapidly, the elderly more slowly. Exercise, digestion, emotional stress, disease conditions, some drugs, stimulants, heat and cold all affect the number of times a person breathes per minute.

Abnormal Respirations

- *Stertorous respirations:* The person makes abnormal noises like a snoring sound.
- *Shallow respirations:* The person breathes using mostly abdominal muscles.

- *Irregular respirations:* The person's breathing changes and the rate of the rise and fall of the chest is not steady.
- *Cheyne-Stokes respirations:* The person's breathing is slow and shallow; then the respirations become faster and deeper until they reach a peak. Then the client breathes shallowly again. Breathing may stop for periods of about 10 seconds. This type of breathing may be caused by certain diseases. It frequently occurs before death.

Procedure: Measuring Respirations

1. Assemble the equipment: watch with a second hand, pad and pencil.
2. Hold the client's wrist as if you were measuring his pulse. Count the client's respirations without the client knowing it. You can do this immediately after counting his pulse.
3. If the client is a child, is restless, or has been crying, wait until he is quiet before counting his respirations. You may count the respirations of someone when he is asleep.
4. One rise and fall of the client's chest counts as one respiration. If you cannot clearly see the chest move, fold the client's arm across his chest and feel the chest move.
5. Check the position of the second hand on the watch. Count "one" when you see the chest rising. Keep counting for a full minute each time the chest rises. Check if your agency permits you to count for 30 seconds and multiply by two.
6. Record the number of respirations. Note whether the respirations are noisy, shallow, labored, or irregular.

Measuring Blood Pressure

Blood pressure is the force of the blood pushing against the walls of the blood vessels. When you take a client's blood pressure, you are measuring the force of the blood pushing through the arteries. The heart contracts as it pumps the blood into the arteries. This pressure is called the *systolic pressure*. When the heart relaxes, the pressure is lowest and is called *diastolic pressure*. You will be measuring both pressures.

In young healthy adults below 40 years old, the normal pressure range is 140 millimeters of mercury systolic and below 90 millimeters of mercury diastolic. These figures are written as follows

$$140/90 \text{ or } \frac{140}{90} = \text{systolic}$$
$$= \text{diastolic}$$

In adults over 40 years old, 160/90 or less is considered normal.

When a person's blood pressure is higher than normal, it is referred to as *hypertension*. When the blood pressure is lower than normal, it is referred to as *hypotension*. One reading of elevated blood pressure does not mean a person has hypertension. This diagnosis can only be made by a physician after a complete medical evaluation.

A *sphygmomanometer* or blood pressure cuff and a stethoscope are used to measure blood pressure. There are two kinds of blood pressure cuffs: an *aneroid* or *dial type* and a *mercury type*. Both have an inflatable cuff. The cuff is wrapped around the client's arm and inflated with the rubber bulb. When using the mercury type, the measurement is read watching the level of the column of mercury. When reading the aneroid type, the measurement is read by watching the dial.

When you take a client's blood pressure, you are listening to the brachial pulse with the stethoscope and watching the dial or the mercury. As you listen, it is important to note the first tapping sound you hear and then the last sound. Sometimes you will hear a tapping sound and then silence, then a tapping sound again. The true reading is the first sound you hear and the last. Record these two sounds. If you should hear the tapping sound all the way to zero, try and listen for a change in the sounds. Record as follows:

142/60/0
142 = systolic reading–first tapping sound
 60 = diastolic sound–change in sound
  0 = last sound heard

Procedure: Measuring Blood Pressure

1. Assemble the equipment: sphygmomanometer (blood pressure cuff), stethoscope, antiseptic swab, pad and pencil.
2. Have the client resting or sitting quietly.
3. Wipe the ear pieces of the stethoscope with the antiseptic swab.
4. If you are using the mercury-type apparatus, the mercury should be at eye level.
5. The client's arm should be exposed to well above the elbow. The client's arm should be supported either on a bed, a chair, a table, or by your hip with the palm upward.
6. Unroll the cuff, loosen the valve on the bulb, and squeeze the compression bag to be sure it is deflated completely. Wrap the cuff snugly and smoothly around the client's arm above the elbow. Do not wrap

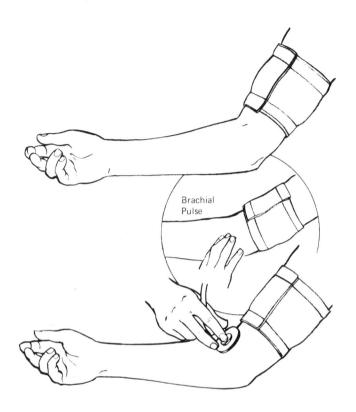

Brachial
Pulse

it so tightly that the client is uncomfortable. Leave the area clear where you will place the stethoscope.

7. With your fingertips, find the client's brachial pulse at the inner side of the arm above the elbow.

Hold your fingers there and inflate the cuff until the pulse disappears. Tighten the thumbscrew of the valve to close it. Turn it clockwise but not too tightly.

Note the reading on the indicator. Quickly deflate the cuff. This is the approximation of the client's systolic reading and is called the *palpated systolic pressure*.

8. Put the ear pieces of the stethoscope into your ears facing forward and place the bell or diaphragm of the stethoscope on the brachial pulse. Hold it snugly but not too tightly. Do not let the stethoscope touch the blood pressure cuff. Hold the stethoscope in place. Inflate the cuff until the dial of mercury is 30 millimeters above the palpated systolic pressure. Open the valve counterclockwise. This allows the air to escape. Let it out slowly until the sound of the pulse comes back. A few seconds must go by without sounds. If you hear pulse sounds immediately, you must stop the procedure, completely deflate the cuff, and reinflate it

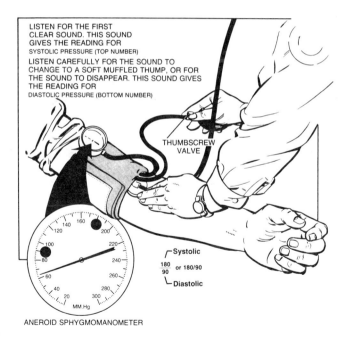

LISTEN FOR THE FIRST
CLEAR SOUND. THIS SOUND
GIVES THE READING FOR
SYSTOLIC PRESSURE (TOP NUMBER)

LISTEN CAREFULLY FOR THE SOUND TO
CHANGE TO A SOFT MUFFLED THUMP, OR FOR
THE SOUND TO DISAPPEAR. THIS SOUND GIVES
THE READING FOR
DIASTOLIC PRESSURE (BOTTOM NUMBER)

THUMBSCREW
VALVE

Systolic
180
90 or 180/90
Diastolic

ANEROID SPHYGMOMANOMETER

to 200 millimeters and again loosen the thumbscrew and listen.

9. Note the calibrations that the pointer or column passes as you hear the first sound. Continue releasing air and note when the sound changes to a faster thud or disappears.

10. Deflate the cuff completely. Remove it from the client's arm. Record your readings.

14

Intake and Output

FLUID BALANCE

Water is essential to human life. Losing one-fifth of the body fluid can cause the body to stop functioning.

Through eating and drinking, the average healthy adult takes in about three and one-half quarts of fluid every 24 hours. This is called *fluid intake*. The *fluid output* is about the same three and one-half quarts a day. When this balance is disrupted, there is said to be a *fluid imbalance*. The fluid may be held in the tissues causing them to swell. This is called *edema*. When the tissues do not hold enough fluid, the body is experiencing *dehydration*.

Fluid is released from the body through

- The kidneys in the form of urine
- The skin in the form of perspiration
- The lungs during breathing
- The intestinal tract

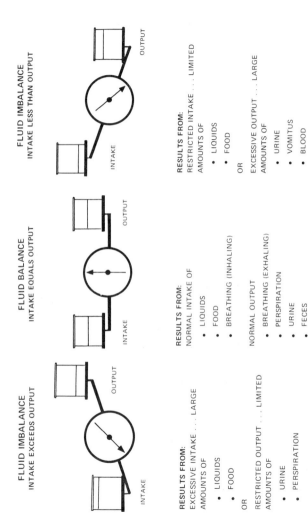

FLUID IMBALANCE
INTAKE EXCEEDS OUTPUT

RESULTS FROM:
EXCESSIVE INTAKE . . . LARGE
AMOUNTS OF
- LIQUIDS
- FOOD

OR

RESTRICTED OUTPUT . . . LIMITED
AMOUNTS OF
- URINE
- PERSPIRATION

FLUID BALANCE
INTAKE EQUALS OUTPUT

RESULTS FROM:
NORMAL INTAKE OF
- LIQUIDS
- FOOD
- BREATHING (INHALING)

NORMAL OUTPUT
- BREATHING (EXHALING)
- PERSPIRATION
- URINE
- FECES

FLUID IMBALANCE
INTAKE LESS THAN OUTPUT

RESULTS FROM:
RESTRICTED INTAKE . . . LIMITED
AMOUNTS OF
- LIQUIDS
- FOOD

OR

EXCESSIVE OUTPUT . . . LARGE
AMOUNTS OF
- URINE
- VOMITUS
- BLOOD
- DRAINAGE
- PERSPIRATION

216

Many things can affect fluid balance:

- Medication
- Exercise
- Weather
- Emotional stress
- Nourishment
- General health

Keeping Records of Fluid Balance

Records are kept of a person's intake and output so that the balance can be monitored and decisions can be made as to the function of the body.

In the United States, we normally use one system for measuring liquids (ounces, pints, quarts, gallons) and a different system for measuring lengths (inches, feet, yards, miles). Scientists use the *metric system* for measuring liquids and lengths. The basic measurement is the *meter* which is longer than a yard. A *centimeter* (c) is 0.01 (one one-hundredth) of a meter or about 0.4 (four tenths) of an inch. A *cubic centimeter* (cc) is a block with each edge 1 centimeter long. If this block was filled with water, it would be a cubic centimeter or, 1 cc.

U.S. CUSTOMARY
LIQUID MEASURE
WITH EQUIVALENT
METRIC MEASUREMENTS

cc = cubic centimeter
ml = milliliter
oz = ounce
1 cc = 1 ml
¼ teaspoon = 1 cc
1 teaspoon = 4 cc
30 cc = 1 oz
60 cc = 2 oz
90 cc = 3 oz
120 cc = 4 oz
150 cc = 5 oz
180 cc = 6 oz
210 cc = 7 oz
240 cc = 8 oz
270 cc = 9 oz
300 cc = 10 oz

500 cc = 1 pint
1000 cc = 1 quart
4000 cc = 1 gallon

pt = pint
qt = quart
gal = gallon

An *intake and output (I&O) record* is often kept in the home near the client's bed. It is totaled every 24 hours. Be sure that everybody in the house understands how to

INTAKE AND OUTPUT SHEET					
Client's Name _____ Date _____					
INTAKE			OUTPUT		
TIME		AMT.	TIME		AMT.
TOTAL			TOTAL		

keep this record so that it will be accurate when you are not there.

A 24 hour intake record is started with the first fluids the client drinks in the morning. However, the first urinary output is considered to be part of the previous day's I&O because the fluid that formed this urine was consumed in the previous 24 hour period. Thus, this first urinary output is discarded. Remember, the first urine recorded is actually the second urinary output of the day.

Fluid Intake

Fluid intake consists of all liquids the client drinks.

A container or measuring cup is used to measure intake and output. If you use a measuring cup *calibrated* with a row of short lines and numbers, you will be able to quickly see the number of ounces and cubic centimeters of the liquid you are measuring. You could also use a baby bottle. It is important to use one container to measure intake and a separate one to measure output. You will be measuring how much liquid a container holds and how much the client drinks. Be sure you are accurate and keep these two numbers separate.

Think about the fluids each time you bring the client something to drink. When measuring the fluid intake, you will have to note the difference between the amount the client drinks, the capacity of the container, and the amount the client leaves in the container.

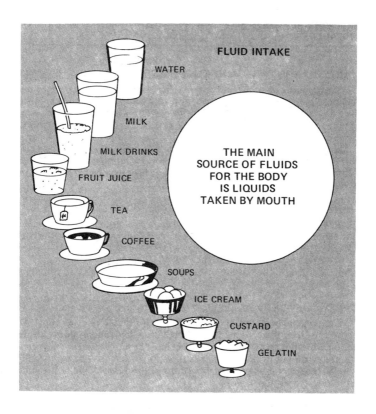

FLUID INTAKE

WATER

MILK

MILK DRINKS

FRUIT JUICE

TEA

COFFEE

SOUPS

ICE CREAM

CUSTARD

GELATIN

THE MAIN SOURCE OF FLUIDS FOR THE BODY IS LIQUIDS TAKEN BY MOUTH

Tell the client his intake and output are being measured. Encourage the client to keep as much of the record as possible. Record the fluid intake as soon as the client consumes the fluid.

It is always easier when the intake and the output are measured using the same unit of measures.

Procedure: Measuring the Capacity of a Serving Container

1. Assemble the equipment: complete set of dishes and glasses used by the client, measuring cup, water, pad and pencil.
2. Fill the first container with water.
3. Pour this water into the measuring cup. Look at the level of water and determine the amount in cc's. Write this information on the paper. Repeat this process until you have a list of the fluid capacity of the cups and dishes the client usually uses.

Procedure: Determining the Amount of Fluid Consumed

1. Assemble the equipment: measuring cup, pad and pencil, leftover liquids in their serving containers.
2. Pour the leftover liquid into the measuring cup. Determine the amount of fluid in cc's.
3. From your list, note the amount of liquid the serving container holds when full.
4. Subtract the leftover amount from the full container. This figure is the amount of fluid the client has consumed. Immediately write down this number on the intake side of the I&O sheet.

Fluid Output

Fluid output is the sum total of all fluids that come out of the body. Most fluid is discharged from the body as urine. Output also includes drainage from a wound, blood, excessive perspiration, and vomitus.

Tell the client his output is being measured and that he must use a commode, bedpan or urinal when he has to urinate. Ask the client not to put the toilet paper into the bedpan. Provide a plastic bag for this and dispose of the tissue in the toilet. Ask the client not to move his bowels while urinating if possible.

Procedure: Measuring Urinary Output

1. Assemble the equipment: bedpan or covered urinal, measuring container, pad and pencil.
2. Pour the urine into the measuring container. Determine the amount of fluid in cc's. Remember the amount.
3. Pour the urine into the toilet. Rinse the container and the urinal or bedpan. Pour this water into the toilet also. Put away all the equipment.
4. Wash your hands. Record the amount of urine and its character, color, and odor.

Measuring Output from an Indwelling Catheter

Some clients have a *catheter* inserted into their urinary bladder by the doctor or nurse. The catheter may also be called a *Foley catheter*. It drains all the client's urine into a plastic urine container, which hangs below the level of the urinary bladder. Empty this container and measure the amount of urine. Record this amount. Do this whenever the container is full and before the end of your working shift. The measurement should not be taken from the soft, expandable, plastic container. Transfer the urine to a measuring container.

Procedure: Emptying a Urinary Collection Bag from an Indwelling Catheter

1. Assemble the equipment: measuring container, paper towels, pad and pencil.
2. Protect the floor with paper towels. Open the drain at the bottom of the plastic urine container and let the urine run into the measuring container. Close the drain. Be sure the urine or the drain does not touch the floor. Keep the tubing from the bag off the floor.
3. Determine the amount of fluid in cc's. Remember it.

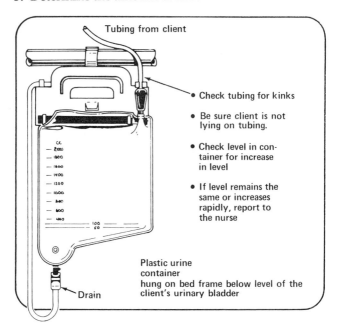

Tubing from client

- Check tubing for kinks
- Be sure client is not lying on tubing.
- Check level in container for increase in level
- If level remains the same or increases rapidly, report to the nurse

Plastic urine container
hung on bed frame below level of the client's urinary bladder

Drain

4. Pour the urine into the toilet. Rinse the container. Pour this water into the toilet. Put away all the equipment.
5. Wash your hands. Record the amount of urine and its character, color,and odor.

Fluid Output from the Incontinent Client

If the client is *incontinent*, record this on the output side of the I&O sheet each time the bed is wet. Even if the urine cannot be measured, it will be obvious that the client's kidneys are functioning. Record the time; the size of the wet area; and the color, odor, and character of the urine.

Measuring Fluids Other than Urine

Vomitus and diarrhea should also be measured according to the procedure for measuring urine. Be sure to indicate the type of fluid you are measuring.

When recording the drainage from a wound or heavy perspiration, indicate the following:

- What was wet
- How wet: damp, dripping, and so forth
- The size of the wet area
- The time
- The color
- The odor
- The character

FORCING AND RESTRICTING FLUIDS

A client who must have more fluids added to his intake is told to *force fluids*. This client often needs encouragement to drink. Be sure you know how much fluid the client is to have within a 24-hour period.

- Show enthusiasm and be cheerful when offering fluids.
- Provide a variety of fluids that the client prefers.
- Offer both hot and cold liquids.
- Offer liquids in small amounts.
- Record the amount of fluids accurately.

Some clients must *restrict* their fluid intake. This means they have a limited amount of fluid they may consume in a 24-hour period. Be sure you know the amount. Be calm and reassuring when offering fluids and when explaining the reason for withholding them.

- Alternate different fluids as permitted.
- Show enthusiasm and be cheerful when offering fluids.
- Provide a variety of fluids the client prefers.
- Offer both hot and cold liquids.
- Offer liquids in small amounts.
- Record the amount of fluids accurately.
- If the restriction is severe, the client may be permitted to suck on ice.

15

Specimen Collection

SPECIMEN COLLECTION

One of the body's normal functions is to regularly get rid
of waste products. When these products are tested in the
laboratory, changes in bodily functions can be detected.
Specimens are samples of bodily waste products that are
collected and sent to the laboratory for examination.

When collecting specimens, use good medical aseptic technique to prevent contamination. Wash your
hands carefully before and after collection. Hand washing before you collect a specimen prevents contamination of the specimen from anything you may have on
your hands. Hand washing after you collect the specimen prevents microorganisms that might be in the specimen from remaining on your hands.

Be sure you

- Know what type of specimen is needed.
- Know when the specimen is to be obtained.
- Have the proper container for the specimen.
- Know when and how it will be sent to the laboratory.

- Know how to store the specimen before it is sent to the laboratory.
- Are accurate in the labeling of the specimen. Include the client's name, address, and age, the correct date and the time you obtain the specimen. Write on the label and attach the label securely to the container.

BE ACCURATE. . .

Print client's name, address

Print clearly so the label can be easily read

Put label on specimen immediately after specimen container has been collected

Type of specimen

Print date and time

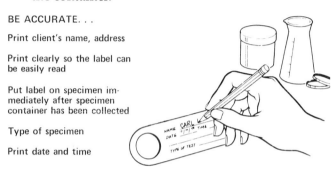

Collecting a Urine Specimen

A *routine urine specimen* is a single sample of urine taken from the client as he voids in the usual way. At times you will be told to take a specimen of the first urine of the day. If you have not been instructed as to when to take the specimen, it may be obtained at any time.

- Prepare the label for the clean container before you pour the urine. Be sure the outside of the container is dry before you put the label on. Indicate if the specimen is obtained from a Foley catheter.
- If possible, have the client void directly into the container. If not, the client should void into a commode, bedpan, or urinal. Transfer the urine to the container.

- If the client is keeping a record of his intake and output, measure the specimen and record the amount.
- Store the specimen in the proper place.

Procedure: Obtaining a Urine Specimen from a Client with a Foley Catheter

1. Assemble the equipment: specimen container and lid, completed label, measuring container, disposable gloves, padding to protect the bed, protective cap or sterile gauze for the drainage tubing.
2. Tell the client a urine specimen is needed. Explain the procedure to him.
3. Place the client in a comfortable position, usually on his back. Spread bed protectors between the client's legs.
4. Disconnect the catheter from the drainage tubing. Allow the urine in the tube to drip into the collection bag. Cap the tubing. Do not allow the catheter to drop. Hold it.
5. Position the end of the catheter over the specimen bottle and allow the urine to drip into the bottle. This may take time. Fill the specimen bottle about half full. If the client is keeping a record of his intake and output and the specimen bottle is not calibrated, collect the urine into a sterile calibrated container, measure it, and then transfer it to the specimen container.
6. Reattach the catheter to the tubing. Make the client comfortable. Clean and put away the equipment. Wash your hands. Store the specimen in the proper place.

A *clean-catch midstream urine specimen* is one that is obtained with as little contamination as possible.

Procedure: Collecting a Midstream Clean-Catch Urine Specimen

1. Assemble the equipment: clean-catch kit or sterilized jar and sterile cleansing solution, sterile gauze, sterile gloves, bedpan or urinal if the client cannot go to the bathroom, wet washcloth and towel, waste bag, completed label.
2. Tell the client a urine specimen is needed. Explain the procedure to him. If possible, the client may obtain the specimen himself.
3. Open the kit. Put on the sterile gloves if you are going to assist the client. If the client is to do the procedure alone, he should wear the gloves. Do not touch the inside of the container or the lid.
4. For female clients:
   a. Separate the folds of the labia and wipe with one towelette or gauze and solution from the front to the back along one labia. Throw away the wipe.
   b. Wipe the opposite labia with the second towelette. Throw it away.
   c. Wipe down the middle using the third towelette. Throw it away.
5. For male clients:
   a. If the male is not circumcised, pull the foreskin of the penis back before cleansing the penis. Hold it back during urination.
   b. Use a circular motion to clean the head of the penis. Use all three towelettes or gauze and sterile solution. Throw each one away after you use it.
6. Ask the client to start urinating into the bedpan or toilet. Then ask the client to stop. Place the sterile urine container under the stream of urine and ask the client to start urinating again. Fill the container one-half full. The remaining urine may be discarded.

7. If the client is keeping a record of his intake and output and the specimen bottle is not calibrated, collect the urine into a sterile calibrated container, measure it, and then transfer it to the specimen container.

8. Make the client comfortable. Clean and put away the equipment. Wash your hands. Store the specimen in the proper place.

Procedure: Collecting Urine from an Infant

1. Assemble the equipment: urine specimen container, plastic disposable infant urine collector, prepared label filling in the time of the specimen when you obtain it.

2. Explain the procedure to the child and his parents. Children who are not yet toilet trained can understand and are more likely to cooperate if they know what to expect. Use language the child understands. The procedure may appear to be uncomfortable, but it does not hurt the child.

3. Take off the child's diaper. Clean the genital area. Be sure the area is dry as the collector bag will not stick if the skin is wet.

4. Remove the outside piece of paper that surrounds the opening of the plastic urine collector. Be sure the skin is not folded under the sticky part of the collector as you apply it. Place the opening of the bag around the male penis or female meatus. Do not cover the rectum or the specimen may be contaminated with fecal matter.

5. Put on the child's diaper. Check every half hour to see if the infant has voided. When there is urine in the collector bag, carefully remove the bag without spilling the urine or hurting the child. Pour the urine into the specimen container.

6. Wash the genital area. Replace the diaper. Make the client comfortable. Clean and put away the equip-

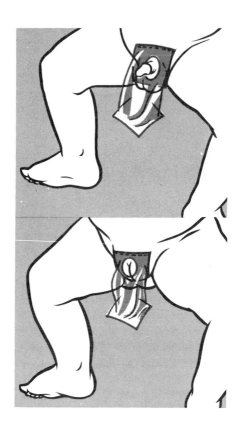

ment. Wash your hands. Store the specimen in the proper place.

Collection of a Stool Specimen

Procedure: Collecting a Stool Specimen

1. Assemble the equipment: bedpan, stool container, completed label, wooden tongue depressor, washcloth and towel.

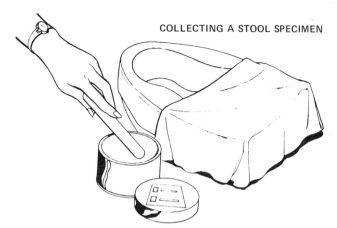

2. Explain the procedure to the client. Have the client move his bowels in the bedpan. If the client is unable to use the bedpan, place several layers of toilet tissue in the bottom of the toilet and have the client move his bowels on the paper. This way you will be able to obtain the specimen easily.

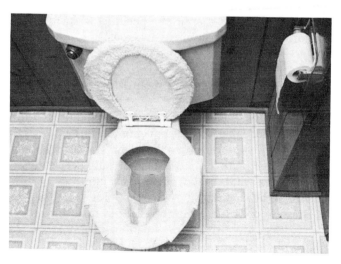

3. Ask the client not to urinate into the bedpan or the toilet and not to put toilet tissue into either. Provide a plastic or paper bag to dispose of the toilet tissue temporarily. Then discard the tissue into the toilet.
4. After the client has moved his bowels, take the bedpan into the bathroom. Wash your hands. Offer the client a washcloth and towel. Make him comfortable.
5. Using a wooden tongue depressor, take a small amount of stool from the bedpan and place it into the stool specimen container. Cover the container. Wrap the depressor in a piece of toilet tissue and dispose of it in a plastic bag. Empty the remaining feces into the toilet and flush it.
6. Clean the bedpan and return it to its proper place. Wash your hands.

Collecting a Sputum Specimen

Sputum is the substance collected from a client's lungs. It contains saliva, mucus, and sometimes blood or pus. The best time to collect a sputum specimen is early in the morning, right after the client awakens.

Procedure: Collecting a Sputum Specimen

1. Assemble the equipment: sputum container and lid, completed label, tissues, paper or plastic bag.
2. Explain the procedure to the client. The client should rinse his mouth if breakfast has already been eaten. If the client wants oral hygiene, assist him.
3. Assist the client to sit or lie on his side. Give him the sputum container. Ask the client to take three deep breaths. After the third breath, ask him to exhale deeply and cough. The client should be able to bring

up some sputum and spit it directly into the container. Saliva is not adequate.

4. Cover the container immediately. Offer the client oral hygiene. Make the client comfortable. Wash your hands. Be sure to store the specimen properly.

16

Special Procedures

ASSISTING WITH MEDICATIONS

Medication is prescribed by a physician, dispensed by a pharmacist, and *administered* or given without client assistance by a nurse or physician. These professionals are licensed by the state to perform their duties. Failure to stay within the law can result in legal action ending in a fine, the revoking of a license, or even jail. Since you are *not* licensed, you are *not* permitted to administer medication. You are, however, permitted to assist your client as he takes his own medications. When you assist the client, he shares the responsibility of giving the medication.

Prescription drugs are prescribed by a physician and cannot be bought without a prescription. Over-the-counter drugs can be bought without a prescription. You will not administer either type of drug.

You will be instructed concerning your responsibilities relating to the client's medication. You will also have to know some basic information.

THE FIVE RIGHTS OF MEDICATION

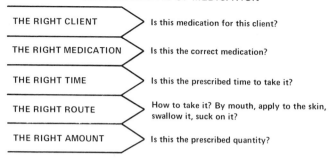

THE RIGHT CLIENT	Is this medication for this client?
THE RIGHT MEDICATION	Is this the correct medication?
THE RIGHT TIME	Is this the prescribed time to take it?
THE RIGHT ROUTE	How to take it? By mouth, apply to the skin, swallow it, suck on it?
THE RIGHT AMOUNT	Is this the prescribed quantity?

You should ask about the side effects of the medications. If the client tells you he suffers from any of them, report it to your supervisor immediately. Also report

- If your client is not taking the medication exactly as it has been prescribed
- If your client is taking medication that your supervisor is not aware of
- Does not know why a drug is being taken
- Has nausea, vomiting, diarrhea, itching, difficulty breathing, a rash or hives soon after taking medication
- Has changes in orientation, concentration , memory, or mood soon after taking medication
- Is confusing his medication

Medication Storage

As you orient yourself to the client's home, notice how he stores his medication. If you notice that medications are stored improperly or unsafely, discuss it with the client or his family. If you cannot do this, discuss the problem with your supervisor so that the two of you can plan how to change the situation.

- Clients save medication and often self-medicate themselves. This is a dangerous practice. Report it if you notice it.
- Many medications have similar names. Store each one separately to avoid accidentally picking up the wrong one.
- Do not assist a client in taking medication from an unlabeled container.
- Do not change the place your client stores his medications.
- Keep medications away from children and confused, forgetful adults.
- Dispose of medications by flushing them down a toilet or pouring them down a drain. Dispose of old medications so no one can eat or otherwise misuse them.

Procedure: Assisting a Client with Medication

1. Assemble the equipment: medication, spoon, water or juice, dressing if medication is applied to the skin, tissue or cotton balls.
2. Remind the client it is time to take his medication. Check the five rights of medication. Put the medication within reach of the client. Loosen the top of the bottle or tubes.
3. Assist the client as necessary.
   a. Oral medication: Hold the client's hand; assist him with liquids.
   b. Ointments: Assist the client as needed with medication and dressings.
   c. Eye drops: Guide the client's hand, wipe excess liquid or ointment from under the eye, from the nose and other areas.
4. Make the client comfortable. Put the medication in its proper place. Wash your hands.

Assisting a Client with Oxygen Therapy

Oxygen is considered a medication. All the rules and responsibilities that apply to you while you are assisting a client with medication apply to you while you are assisting a client with oxygen. After oxygen is prescribed by the physician, it is delivered in a tank to the house. The tank my look like a vacuum cleaner or a piece of furniture, or it may be a big green tank. The company that delivers it is responsible for refilling it, servicing the equipment, and teaching the client how to use the equipment.

Oxygen is dispensed from the tank to the client through a tube. The tube fits onto a mask, a nasal cannula, or a catheter. The physician prescribes the route. Oxygen is very drying, so a nebulizer filled with water or medication is usually attached to the tank. The oxygen passes through the water and takes on moisture before it goes to the client.

A *nasal catheter* is a piece of tubing that is longer than a cannula. It is inserted through the client's nostril into the back of his mouth. The nasal catheter is used when the client must have additional oxygen at all times. The catheter is fastened to the client's forehead or cheek with a piece of tape.

Nasal cannulas are inserted into a client's nostrils. The small plastic tubes are held in place by an elastic band around the client's head.

A *face mask* is used when the client must have a large amount of oxygen. It is secured by an elastic band around the client's head.

Your responsibilities include the following:

- Put up a "No Smoking" sign in the room the client uses. Enforce this rule.
- Report to your supervisor if the client does not use the oxygen as it has been prescribed.

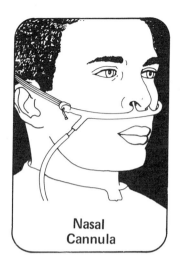

Nasal Cannula

- Use cotton bedclothes to decrease static electricity.
- Do not use electric shavers or hair dryers while the oxygen is running. Keep plugs out of the wall sockets while the oxygen is running. Pulling a plug from the outlet could cause a spark which in turn could cause an explosion.

OXYGEN FACE MASK

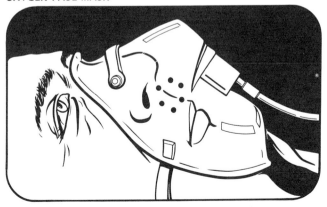

- Do not use candles or open flames in the room.
- Avoid combing the client's hair while the oxygen is on. A spark of electricity from the hair could cause an explosion.
- Do not change the settings on the oxygen tank.
- If oxygen is used, do not allow smoking in the client's room even if the oxygen is shut off.
- Be sure the oxygen is used on the prescribed setting. If this is not being done, report to your supervisor.
- Help the client and his family set realistic short-term goals day by day.
- Assist the client in finding some activities to occupy spare time: small meaningful chores or entertainment that is enjoyable. Some clients enjoy radio, television, tapes, or newspapers. Most clients are unable to concentrate for long periods of time, so activities should be short.

CHANGING NONSTERILE DRESSINGS

Bandages that do not require sterile technique are called *nonsterile dressings*. When you change a dressing, always note the color, odor, amount, and the consistency of the *drainage* on the old dressing. Also note how big the wound is and the condition of the skin surrounding the wound. Note any change in the wound since you last saw it.

Example of Charting Following a Dressing Change

7/3/86 Dressing changed on Mrs. C's right thigh at 10 A.M. Old dressing has light red drainage, 25 cent size, no odor. Wound 5 cent size. Surrounding skin has several small red raised areas. Clean dressing applied. Tape not

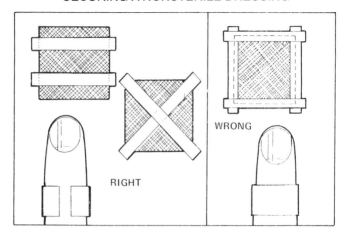

RIGHT

WRONG

applied to red areas. Called supervisor to report. Mary Jones H/HHA

CARE OF AN INDWELLING CATHETER

The urinary catheter is made of plastic or rubber and is inserted by the nurse or physician through the client's urethra into the urinary bladder. A catheter may be used (1) when a client is unable to urinate naturally, (2) to measure the amount of urine left in the bladder after a client has urinated naturally, or (3) to keep an incontinent client dry.

A catheter may be used once, or it may be kept in place for several days or weeks. A catheter that is left in place is called an *indwelling catheter* or *Foley catheter* and has a special balloon that is inflated with water or air to keep it in place. The catheter is attached to a drainage bag or container secured to the bed frame lower than the client's bladder. This collection system is a closed sys-

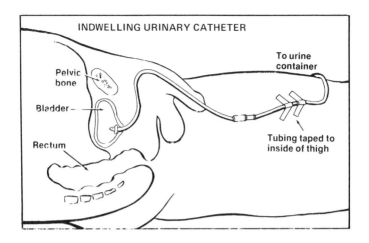

INDWELLING URINARY CATHETER

Pelvic bone

Bladder

Rectum

To urine container

Tubing taped to inside of thigh

tem, which means it is never opened except when the urine is emptied from the collection bag. Most clients who have catheters keep records of their intake and output. Be sure to note the amount of urine you empty from the collection bag.

A leg bag is a small bag worn the client's leg when he is up and active. It cannot be worn when the client is lying down. Empty it frequently.

Secure the catheter to the client's inner thigh to prevent it from pulling. You may use tape or special straps if they are available. Empty the collection bag frequently. There are many types of bags. If you are not sure how to use one, ask for assistance.

All catheters should be secured to the client's inner thigh to prevent pulling. You may use tape or special straps.

Catheters drain by *straight drainage*. This means the tube from the bed to the bag must be kept straight to prevent urine backing up into the client's bladder or kidneys. The rest of the tubing is kept in the bed. The bag goes with the client when he gets out of bed. Always

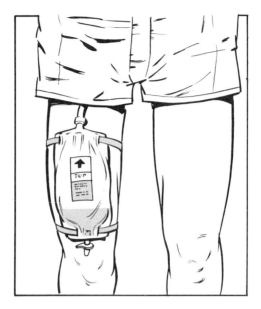

keep it lower than the bladder and maintain the straight drainage. Be sure there are no kinks in the tubing or that the client is not lying or sitting on the tubing. Keep it clean of fecal matter and mucus.

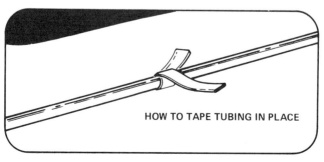

HOW TO TAPE TUBING IN PLACE

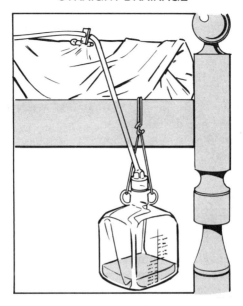

Report to your supervisor if

- The level of urine has not increased in the collection bag
- You notice blood or sediment in the bag or the catheter
- The client feels his bladder is full or if urine leaks around the catheter

Procedure: Catheter Care

This procedure may be incorporated into the morning bath routine. Be sure you use clean water.

1. Assemble your equipment: basin of water, mild soap or cleansing solution, washcloth or gauze pads, paper or plastic bag for waste, disposable gloves.

2. Tell the client you are going to provide catheter care. Position the client on his back so that the catheter and urinary meatus are exposed. Put on gloves.

3. Wash the urinary meatus gently without pulling on the catheter. Wipe one way and not back and forth. Observe the meatus for redness, swelling, or discharge.

4. Remove your gloves. Dry the area. Apply lotion or cornstarch to the thighs.

5. Be sure the client is safe and comfortable. Clean and put away the equipment. Wash your hands.

Procedure: Changing a Catheter from a Straight Drainage Bag to a Leg Bag

1. Assemble the equipment: leg bag and straps, alcohol wipes or antiseptic solution, sterile cover for straight drainage tubing or sterile 4 by 4, a bed protector.

2. Tell the client you are going to put on the leg bag. Expose the end of the catheter and the drainage tubing. Put a bed protector under this area.

3. Disconnect the drainage tubing from the catheter and allow it to drain. Put a sterile cover on the end and place it out of the way, but not on the floor.

4. Wipe the attachment tube of the leg bag with an alcohol swab and insert it into the catheter. Secure the leg bag to the client's thigh.

5. Be sure the client is safe and comfortable. Wash your hands.

External Urinary Drainage

External urinary drainage is used when a male client is incontinent of urine. It should not be kept on for more

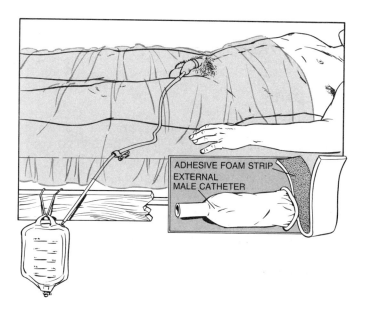

ADHESIVE FOAM STRIP
EXTERNAL
MALE CATHETER

than 24 hours at a time and should be removed to clean the penis and inspect the tissue.

Procedure: External Urinary Drainage

1. Assemble the equipment: external urinary drainage system, tape or strap to secure condom to penis, soap and water, towel.
2. Tell the client you are going to put on an external urinary drainage system. Position the client so that the penis is exposed. Wash the penis well and dry the area thoroughly.
3. Roll the condom onto the entire length of the penis and secure it in place. Be careful not to make it too tight.
4. Attach the catheter to the other end of the condom. Set up the straight drainage and secure the tubing.

5. Be sure the client is safe and comfortable. Clean and put away the equipment. Wash your hands.

CAST CARE

Clients who have broken a bone or sprained or strained a muscle may have a *cast* or *splint* on the injured body part to immobilize it as it heals. Casts and splints are temporary and are removed when the physician feels it is appropriate. The casts may be plaster, fiber glass, or plastic. It is normal for a plaster cast to feel warm while it is drying and hardening.

Call your supervisor if you notice any of the following:

- Pain from the cast
- Numbness or tingling of the toes or fingers
- Discoloration of toes or fingers
- Swelling of the limb at the edge of the cast
- Rough or cracked edges of the cast
- Loosely fitted cast
- Discoloration of the cast

ASSISTING WITH OSTOMY CARE

The creation of an *ostomy* is a surgical procedure which creates an opening for the release of wastes through the abdomen. The opening is called a *stoma*. This operation is necessary when the colon or urinary system is diseased or injured. Sometimes the surgery is permanent and sometimes it is temporary.

Colostomy is an opening into the colon.

Ileostomy is an opening into the ileum.

Ureterostomy is an opening into the ureter.

A person with an ostomy must wear an appliance to collect the matter released through the stoma. This collection bag is held on with special paste and/or a belt. Some appliances are used several times and some are thrown away after one use.

You will be asked to assist the client with the changing of the appliance and the cleansing of the skin surrounding the stoma. Ask to be shown the procedure the

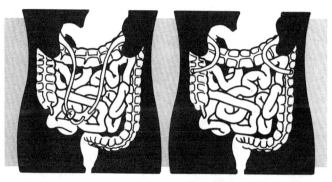

Ileal Conduit   Bilateral Cutaneous Ureterostomy

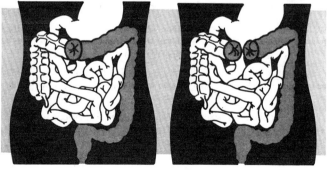

Transverse (Single Barrel)   Transverse (Double Barrel)

client will follow and then do not deviate from it. There are many types of appliances and many products. It is important to follow the procedure appropriate for your client's appliance.

If your client is instructed to *irrigate* his colostomy, you may be asked to assist with this procedure which is like giving a small enema through the stoma. Do not do so, however, until you have been specifically instructed.

There are ostomies through which a client can take nourishment: *gastrostomy*, *duodenostomy*, and a *jejunostomy*. These openings are kept open by the presence of a screw top or a tube. You will be shown how to assist with the care of these.

ASSISTING A CLIENT HAVING A SEIZURE

A *seizure* is caused by an abnormality within the central nervous system. They can be caused by a head injury or can be present from birth. Seizures can usually be controlled by medication. People with epilepsy, or seizures, can lead very productive lives if they are able to follow their medical regime. When they become ill, however, or have undue stress, their medication might have to be readjusted.

Some clients know they are going to have a seizure. This is called an *aura*. An aura may be a smell or sensation that always occurs before a seizure. The client has no memory of the seizure. There are two types of seizures:

grand mal seizure: total stiffness of the body followed by a jerking motion of the muscles. Usually the client becomes unconscious and may or may not become incontinent. This lasts for several minutes.

petit mal seizure: may appear as though the client is daydreaming. There may be some quivering of the muscles and the eyes may roll backward. This lasts for about 30 seconds.

The best action to take when a client has a seizure is to protect him from hurting himself and to protect him from the stares of others. Ask the client and the family what they usually do when a seizure starts. They may have a padded tongue blade or a belt they place in the client's mouth to prevent him from biting his tongue. *Do not pry the mouth open after the seizure has started. Do not put your hands in the client's mouth.* After the seizure, allow the client to sleep or relax. If he has been incontinent, help him with the cleaning process.

TESTING URINE FOR SUGAR AND ACETONE

There are many ways to test the urine. Read the instructions on the package of testing material and ask the client, family and your supervisor for instructions.

- How often should you test the urine?
- Where should you record the results?
- What is the usual time of day to test the urine?
- After you have tested the urine, what should you do with the results? Which values indicate a need for you to call your supervisor?

DEEP BREATHING EXERCISES

Deep breathing helps people inhale more air as the lower lobes of the lungs expand. As the air is forcibly exhaled, the client releases more air. This type of breathing exchanges more air than normal breathing.

Clients with lung disease often have to be encouraged to do this since they are not used to breathing with their abdominal muscles. This type of breathing may cause the client to cough.

A physical therapist will set up the deep breathing regime for the client. Do not start this procedure until the therapist instructs you.

MAKING NORMAL SALINE

Normal saline is a solution of water and salt. It can be used to wash open areas, to cleanse bedsores, or to irrigate catheters.

Procedure: Making Normal Saline

1. Assemble the equipment: large pot, sterilized 1 quart jar and lid, 2 teaspoons salt; 1 quart water, source of heat (stove, sterno, etc.)
2. Measure 1 quart water into the pot. Add 2 teaspoons salt. Boil covered for ten minutes.
3. Pour into sterilized jar. Cover and allow to cool. The solution may be used up to 48 hours after preparation.

SITZ BATH

A *sitz bath* bathes the perineal area to promote healing, decrease pain, and prompt relaxation of the muscles. The bath can be taken either in a specially designed bath that fits into the toilet or in the bathtub which has had a covered rubber ring placed in it.

- Be sure the water is the correct temperature. It should be comfortable.
- Be sure the client is safe.
- Do not let the client bathe for more than 15 minutes.

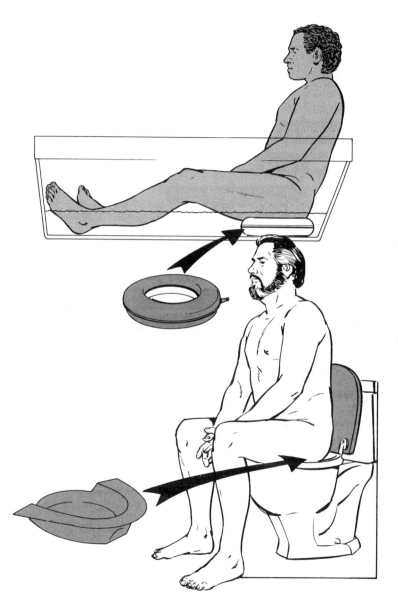

17

Common Diseases

HYPERTENSION

Hypertension or high blood pressure is a treatable chronic disease that is present in about 35 million Americans. Hypertension has been called the "silent killer" because it gives no warning. In the early stages there are no symptoms. As the disease develops, people may complain of headaches, changes in vision, or changes in urinary output. If they consult a physician, obtain medication and change their life style, permanent damage to vital organs would be prevented. Many people, however, do not seek help until they have had a stroke or suffered some permanent organ damage.

All the causes of hypertension are unknown, but people who are apt to have hypertension are those who

- Have a family history of hypertension, heart disease or kidney disease
- Smoke
- Are overweight
- Use a lot of salt in their diet

- Are black
- Eat a large amount of saturated fats

Treatment for hypertension is available, but it must be kept up forever. Just because blood pressure is brought under control, it does not mean the disease has gone away.

- Help the client and his family incorporate the medication regime, diet plan, and exercise schedule into their daily routine.
- If the client or his family has questions, answer him honestly and refer him to his physician for further discussion.
- Report possible side effects of medication. If the client has noticed any change in his activity level or in the way he feels, these changes should be reported to the physician. Medication can be changed or the dosage altered. No medication should be stopped without notifying the prescribing physician.

HEART ATTACK/MYOCARDIAL INFARCTION

A *heart attack* is a general term to describe a sudden damage to the heart. There are many medical reasons people have heart attacks, but they all result in a decrease of blood supply to the heart and possible permanent damage to the heart tissue. This condition, the death of the heart tissue due to loss of blood supply is called a *myocardial infarction* or *MI*. If the amount of tissue damage is small, it may be called a *minor heart attack*. If damage is considerable, it will be called a *massive heart attack*. The ultimate recovery of the injured heart depends on many things:

- Location of the MI
- Age
- Health history
- Sex
- Atherosclerosis

Atherosclerosis is a form of *arteriosclerosis* or hardening of the arteries due to a thickening of the blood vessel walls. This takes place in several steps:

- A fatty streak develops in the vessel.
- A fibrous plaque develops and enlarges over time.
- Sometimes a clot develops.

PLAQUE

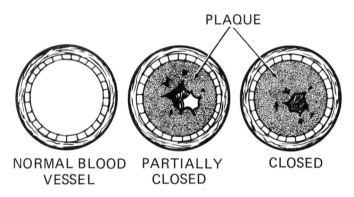

NORMAL BLOOD VESSEL PARTIALLY CLOSED CLOSED

Care from a myocardial infarction is based on

- The type of damage to the heart
- The recovery so far
- The home situation
- The prognosis

Many clients are given an exercise regime. If the client is unable to progress with the exercises or tries to advance too quickly, report this to your supervisor. Some clients completely deny their condition by not following suggestions, medications, or restrictions.

Other clients are so afraid to exert themselves for fear of another heart attack that they become "cardiac cripples." They remove themselves from their family, friends, and work and blame their problems on their medical condition. It is natural for clients to have many of these feelings at various times during their recovery. It is not, however, healthy for them to remain at one extreme or the other.

Clients are very concerned about the effect their heart attack will have upon their sexual activities. If this is of concern, ask your supervisor to discuss this with your client.

Pacemakers

Pacemakers are electrical devices placed in the left upper chest under the skin to regulate the heart rhythm either permanently or on a temporary basis. Be sure you and

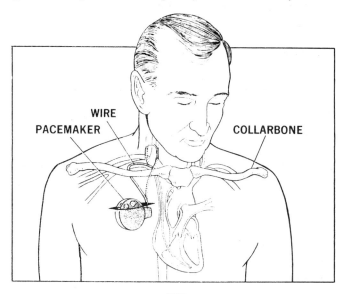

the client know what kind of pacemaker is in place and at what rate it is set. The physician notifies the client when the batteries must be replaced. Pacemakers are monitored in many ways. One of them is by use of the telephone. It is very important that the client performs his particular monitoring procedure at the scheduled time. If he cannot do this, notify your supervisor.

- Electrical appliances may be used around pacemakers. The client with a pacemaker should not be around microwave ovens and some lawn mowers. Detecting devices in airports should be avoided.
- Report the presence of hiccups. This could indicate that a wire is out of place.
- Report if your client's pulse is below the preset level of the pacemaker.
- Report pain or discoloration near the pacemaker.
- Report any complaints of pain, dizziness, edema, shortness of breath, or irregular pulse.

ANGINA

Angina is the brief, temporary pain or heaviness in the chest which results from a lack of oxygen to the heart. Usually, after resting and medication the discomfort disappears. If the angina is allowed to continue without treatment, permanent damage to the heart could result. Changes in the severity, type of pain, or length of pain in your client's angina indicate change in his cardiac status and should be reported to the doctor immediately.

A client has a high risk of angina if he

- Has high blood pressure
- Has high cholesterol
- Smokes cigarettes

- Is overweight
- Has a high stress level

Treatment consists of a regime of medication, control of risk factors, and sometimes even surgery. Since most treatment requires some permanent changes in life style, clients and families often find treatment difficult. Changing the life style of the client also affects the family. Be alert to the support the family offers to the client as these changes are occurring.

- If your client does not maintain the prescribed medication, report it.
- Provide support as the client and his family change their life style to decrease risk factors. This often takes time and great effort.
- Do not dwell on failures. Rather, point out the small successes.

DIABETES

When the body cannot change *carbohydrates* into energy because of an imbalance of *insulin*, the result is the chronic disease known as *diabetes*. The pancreas usually produces insulin on a feedback mechanism. When the body needs insulin following a meal or when extra energy is needed, the pancreas is alerted and it pumps extra insulin into the bloodstream. If the body needs insulin and none is produced, the starches and sugar cannot be converted into energy. The sugar remains in the bloodstream and is eventually excreted in the urine as waste.

There are two types of diabetes. Type I results in the person having to take insulin by injection. In type II, the pancreas produces some insulin but not enough for normal body function. The person may take oral medication or just regulate his diet. In both types of diabetes, the regulation is an important part of the treatment and must be maintained all the time.

Signs and Symptoms of Diabetes

- Fatigue, tiredness
- High blood sugar
- Excessive thirst
- Inflammation which does not heal
- Loss of weight
- Sugar in the urine
- Poor vision
- Frequent and large amounts of urine

Diabetes can be controlled but never cured. People with diabetes can live full and productive lives if they keep a diet and medication regime. Diagnosis of the disease can only be made by a physician following laboratory tests.

Signs and Symptoms of Diabetic Coma (Hyperglycemia/High Blood Sugar-Diabetic Acidosis)

- Loss of appetite
- Nausea and/or vomiting
- Flushed dry skin
- Increased urination
- Dulled senses
- Weakness
- Generalized aches
- Soft eyeballs
- Labored breathing and increased respirations
- Abdominal pains or discomfort
- Increased thirst and parched tongue
- Sweet or fruity odor of the breath
- Upon examination: large amounts of sugar and ketones in the urine and high blood sugar

Signs and Symptoms of Insulin Shock (Hypoglycemia/Low Blood Sugar-Insulin Reaction)

- Excessive perspiration
- Headache
- Faintness, dizziness, weakness
- Hunger
- Tremors, trembling

- Irritability, personality change, nervousness
- Numbness of the tongue and lips
- Sleepiness, coma, unconsciousness
- Blurred or impaired vision
- Upon examination: low blood sugar and no sugar in the urine

Assist the client and his family with

- Medication and diet routine
- Urine testing or finger stick blood testing
- Care of his skin particularly of his feet
- Observations for bruises, difficulty healing or skin irritations
- Maintaining lubricated nonflaky skin
- Keeping doctor's appointments

CEREBROVASCULAR ACCIDENT

The term *cerebrovascular accident* has three important parts:

- *Cerebro*: having to do with the brain
- *Vascular*: having to do with the blood vessels
- *Accident*: something unpredictable and unexpected

A *CVA* or *stroke* occurs when the blood supply to part of the brain is stopped due to a blocked blood vessel. This causes the brain tissue to die. Since each part of the brain controls a different function, the result of the CVA depends on which blood vessel is blocked and which brain center is destroyed. The result of the CVA may be paralysis, loss of vision, or loss of speech; but the cause of the problem is the disruption of nerve impulses from the brain to the body part.

Sometimes when a vessel is blocked, the surrounding blood vessels take over and supply the injured part of the brain. This is called *collateral circulation*. In this case the damage may not be as great.

Causes of CVA

- A blood clot can form elsewhere in the body and travel to the brain and lodge in a small vessel. This is called an *embolus*.
- A blood clot can form in the brain and remain there. This is called a *thrombus*.
- *Plaque* can accumulate in the blood vessels and eventually close them.
- A blood vessel can burst causing a *hemorrhage*.

Assist the client as follows:

- Help families adjust. Clients may live with this condition for 30 years. Families often have difficulties adjusting to the new dependent role of the client.
- Follow the exercise and medication regimes as they have been prescribed. If the family or the client does not adhere to it, report this. Work out a system so that a careful accurate record is kept.
- Assist the family and client with maintaining a safe environment. Help the client set realistic goals for activity.
- Point out the positive aspects of the client's abilities.
- Use simple instructions and words that are familiar to the client.

Be alert

- For changes in his condition

- For observations that may indicate he is regaining some motion or speech
- For stress in the family as they care for the client

ARTHRITIS

Arthritis means inflammation and destruction of the joint. This can be due to an allergy, injury, or infection. Sometimes, the cause is not known. There are over 100 types of arthritis. The most common are

> *Osteoarthritis*: This is the most common type and most commonly seen in the elderly. The joints and their linings wear out with continual use causing the bones to rub together and causing pain every time the joint moves.

> *Rheumatoid*: This is a crippling, chronic disease affecting all connective tissue usually starting in the joints. It often starts in childhood or early adulthood and affects three times more women than men.

OSTEOARTHRITIS—A NORMAL JOINT AND A DISEASED JOINT

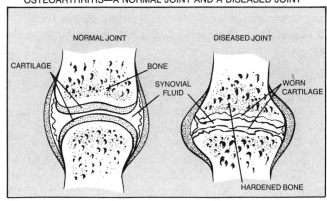

Gout: This disease is most common among men. Uric acid crystals build up in the blood and lodge in the joints causing inflammation and pain. All joints can be affected but the big toe is the most common site.

Ankylosing Spondylitis: This starts usually before the age of 35, most commonly in men and only attacks the spine, shoulders, and hips.

Arthritis is a chronic disease that will be with the client forever. Treatment allows these people to maintain fairly normal active lives.

- Help the client to establish a routine that is safe, and efficient and encourages independence. Balance exercise and rest.
- Assist with the client's medication regime.
- Notice and report changes in activity level, deviations from prescribed regimes, and any reactions to medications.

CANCER

Cancer or *malignancy* is a tumor made up of cells that have changed from normal to abnormal. The course of the disease depends on

- Location of the tumor
- Type of tumor
- When the cancer is discovered
- Type of treatment available
- General health and age of the client

The spread of cancer cells from one area to another is called *metastisis*. The first site is called the primary site and the metastisis is called the secondary site.

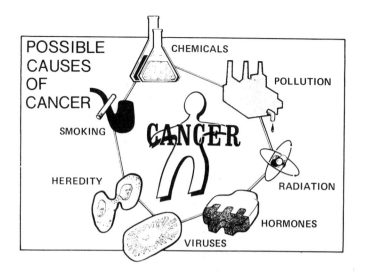

POSSIBLE CAUSES OF CANCER

CHEMICALS

POLLUTION

SMOKING

CANCER

HEREDITY

RADIATION

HORMONES

VIRUSES

The only way to know if a tumor is malignant or not is to have a small piece of tissue examined in a laboratory. This procedure is called a *biopsy*. If the tumor is not *malignant*, it is said to be *benign*.

Treatment varies from client to client and disease to disease. Follow the regime prescribed for your client. The client may have surgery, chemotherapy and/or radiation treatments. Each person reacts differently to the treatments. Some clients get nauseated, some lose their hair. Some have no reaction at all. Be alert to your client's reactions and report them so that medication or diet changes can be prescribed.

Cancer is not contagious. Encourage family and friends to spend time with the client and show their support. Provide an atmosphere in which the client can ask questions and receive honest answers. Do not lie. If the client asks a question which you cannot or should not answer, explain you do not have the complete an-

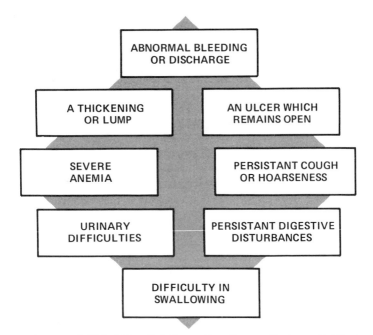

WARNING SIGNS OF CANCER

swer but you will get it. Then discuss the answer with the family or your supervisor.

Some families choose not to tell the client about his diagnosis. Although you may not agree with this, you must adhere to the wishes of the family.

ALZHEIMER'S DISEASE

Alzheimer's disease is the major cause of mental deterioration among the over 65 population. Although some victims of this disease are institutionalized, most are cared for in their home. This disease is chronic, progressive, and ultimately renders the person totally dependent upon others. There is no known cure. The progression varies in each client. Each stage may last several years.

Institutionalization may or may not take place. Each family copes in a different manner. Be supportive to the family as they make the decision that is best for them.

The care of a family member with this disease is very draining upon a family as it takes money and time to provide a safe atmosphere. Since these clients require progressive care over many, many years, families are often resentful of this burden. Often family members must stop working in order to care for their family member. Having a person with Alzheimer's disease in the house always changes a family's life style. Many caregivers become isolated from friends and other members of the family. Do not be judgmental of the actions or words of family members but rather seek additional support for them. Support differs in each state and each community.

Stage I: The client is able to cover up his memory loss, decreased speech, and agitation. Many clients sense the change but are unable to verbalize it. They are embarrassed, depressed, and withdrawn. Families often label these clients forgetful or disinterested.

Stage II. The client may stop speaking, wander, repeat meaningless movements, put all types of things in his mouth. There may be a change in appetite and the client may start to pace.

Stage III. Continual supervision is necessary. The client must be fed and coaxed to eat. He may finally become unresponsive.

Each client has a slightly different care routine. Help the family adapt the plan to best fit their life style, capabilities, and financial resources. The maintenance of a routine in a quiet, unstressed environment is important in caring for these clients. Do not change the routine unless it is necessary.

- Be alert for the safety of the clients and the family.
- Be alert for changes in the client's abilities and responses. Report them as soon as they are noticed.
- Maintain a toileting and personal hygiene routine. This prevents skin breakdown and possible infections.
- Offer small nutritious meals and sips of water. Be alert for signs of dehydration.
- Monitor the client's sleep patterns. Report changes.
- Be supportive of family members and their needs. Observe changes in family dynamics. Report them. Be alert to family tensions. Often by discussing them, a solution can be found.
- Be alert to your feelings as you care for the client over a long period of time. If you need support, ask your supervisor.
- Encourage the caregiver to leave the house while you are there.

CHRONIC OBSTRUCTIVE PULMONARY DISEASE

Chronic obstructive pulmonary disease (COPD) is a term referring to all diseases that cause irreversible damage to the lungs over a period of time. Effects of COPD are the following:

- Lungs cannot expand, remove oxygen from the air, or exchange it with wastes and carbon dioxide from the body.

- Most clients are susceptible to infection.
- All exercise is difficult. Eating is difficult, and speaking is often kept at a minimum.
- Behavior may be unusual due to high levels of carbon dioxide and other gases in the blood stream. When these blood gases are corrected, behavior returns to normal.
- Chests actually change in shape in an effort to provide a larger area for the lungs to expand.
- As breathing becomes more difficult, oxygen and other machines may be necessary. Some clients require tracheostomies to breathe and feeding tubes to provide nourishment.

As with other chronic diseases, having a family member with COPD affects all members of the family. As the client becomes more dependent, the caregiver becomes more and more isolated. Family relationships become strained because the client is unable to speak or interact with his family. Visitors may stop coming. Finally when the care becomes very time consuming, the caregiver may have to give up a job to stay at home.

You will be able to assist the primary caregiver. Encourage the caregiver to leave the house and pursue other interests when you are there.

- Maintain the schedule and medication regime the primary caregiver has established.
- Report all changes in the client's status and activity level.
- Offer small, nutritious meals. The sense of taste is often diminished so discuss the meals with the client. Do not introduce new foods unless you have discussed it first. If there is a fluid restriction, maintain it.

Index